Emergency Management
of the
Pediatric Patient

CASES, ALGORITHMS, EVIDENCE

**Be prepared for any emergency with
the Emergency Management series**

- Features clinical case scenarios of real-life emergency situations with questions that ask the reader to think critically through management decisions at every step
- Highlights literature and evidence that have molded EM clinical practice
- Includes pocket-sized card with algorithms for quick reference of protocols

*Emergency Management of the Coding Patient:
Cases, Algorithms, Evidence*
A step-by-step guide to the clinical and leadership skills needed to run a hospital code with review of ACLS protocols

*Emergency Management of the Pediatric Patient:
Cases, Algorithms, Evidence*
A must-have manual detailing effective strategies for initial stabilization and treatment of the critical pediatric patient including PALS review

*Emergency Management of the Trauma Patient:
Cases, Algorithms, Evidence*
A practical resource covering emergency care of trauma patients with a complete review of ATLS protocols

Emergency Management of the Pediatric Patient

CASES, ALGORITHMS, EVIDENCE

Kimball A. Prentiss, MD

Chief Pediatric Resident
Massachusetts General Hospital for Children
Boston, Massachusetts

Nathan W. Mick, MD

Director
Pediatric Emergency Medicine
Maine Medical Center
Portland, Maine

Brian M. Cummings, MD

Fellow in Pediatric Critical Care
Massachusetts General Hospital
Boston, Massachusetts

Michael R. Filbin, MD

Attending Physician
Department of Emergency Medicine
Massachusetts General Hospital
Clinical Instructor, Harvard Medical School
Boston, Massachusetts

Series Founder and Editor: Michael R. Filbin, MD

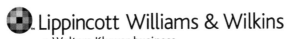

a Wolters Kluwer business
Philadelphia · Baltimore · New York · London
Buenos Aires · Hong Kong · Sydney · Tokyo

Acquisitions Editor: Donna Balado
Managing Editor: Selene Steneck
Marketing Manager: Jennifer Kuklinski
Production Editor: Julie Montalbano
Design Coordinator: Doug Smock
Compositor: International Typesetting and Composition
Printer: Courier—Courier Kendalville

Copyright © 2007 Kimball A. Prentiss

351 West Camden Street
Baltimore, MD 21201

530 Walnut Street
Philadelphia, PA 19106

The publisher is not responsible (as a matter of product liability, negligence, or otherwise) for any injury resulting from any material contained herein. This publication contains information relating to general principles of medical care that should not be construed as specific instructions for individual patients. Manufacturers' product information and package inserts should be reviewed for current information, including contraindications, dosages, and precautions.

Printed in the United States of America

Library of Congress Cataloging-in-Publication Data

Emergency management of the pediatric patient : cases, algorithms, evidence
/ Kimball A. Prentiss . . . [et al.].
      p. ; cm. – (Emergency management series)
   Includes index.
   ISBN 1-4051-0488-0
 1. Pediatric emergencies–Case studies.   2. Pediatric
emergencies--Problems, exercises, etc.   I. Prentiss, Kimball A.   II.
Emergency management series (Blackwell Pub.)
   [DNLM: 1. Emergency Treatment–methods--Case Reports.   2. Emergency
Treatment--methods--Problems and Exercises.   3. Child–Case Reports.   4.
Child--Problems and Exercises.   5. Infant–Case Reports.   6. Infant--Problems
and Exercises.   WS 18.2 E53 2007]
RJ370.E432 2007
618.92'0025--dc22

                                                    2005033267

The publishers have made every effort to trace the copyright holders for borrowed material. If they have inadvertently overlooked any, they will be pleased to make the necessary arrangements at the first opportunity.

To purchase additional copies of this book, call our customer service department at **(800) 638-3030** or fax orders to **(301) 223-2320.** International customers should call **(301) 223-2300.**

Visit Lippincott Williams & Wilkins on the Internet: *http://www.LWW.com.* Lippincott Williams & Wilkins customer service representatives are available from 8:30 am to 6:00 pm, EST.

06 07 08 09 10
1 2 3 4 5 6 7 8 9 10

Kimball A. Prentiss recently completed her pediatric residency at Massachusetts General Hospital for Children and is currently Chief Resident in pediatrics at MGH. She graduated from Middlebury College and was a biology teacher prior to starting medical school at the University of Massachusetts.

Nathan W. Mick is the Director of Pediatric Emergency Medicine at Maine Medical Center in Portland, Maine. He received a bachelor's degree in biology from the University of Notre Dame and graduated from Duke University School of Medicine. He completed residency training in Emergency Medicine at the Harvard Affiliated Emergency Medicine Residency Program and fellowship training in Pediatric Emergency Medicine at Children's Hospital of Boston. An avid outdoorsman, he enjoys mountain biking, hiking, and snowshoeing.

Brian M. Cummings is a fellow in Pediatric Critical Care at Massachusetts General Hospital. He graduated from Boston College with a B.S. in Biology and attended medical school at the University of Connecticut. He completed his residency training in Pediatrics at the Massachusetts General Hospital for Children and continues to work there as a fellow.

Michael R. Filbin is an attending physician in the Emergency Department at Massachusetts General Hospital. He received a bachelor's degree in aerospace engineering from the University of Washington in Seattle. He worked in manned space flight mission operations at the National Aeronautical and Space Agency (NASA) before graduating from medical school at Baylor College of Medicine in Houston. He completed residency at the Harvard Affiliated Emergency Medicine Residency Program in Boston where he now practices and teaches.

Preface

Emergency Management of the Pediatric Patient is part of a new and unique three-book review series that emphasizes case-, algorithm-, and evidence-based learning. The other two books in this series are *Emergency Management of the Trauma Patient* and *Emergency Management of the Coding Patient*.

Emergency Management of the Pediatric Patient: Cases, Algorithms, Evidence aims to simplify the experience of caring for acutely ill children, predominantly within the emergency department. Each chapter presents a realistic case scenario with multiple-choice questions and answers that lead the reader through the management of the case. The body of each chapter reviews basic information related to the given topic with an emphasis on differential diagnoses and other high yield information that can be applied in the clinical setting. The final and unique aspect of this series is the inclusion of literature reference boxes that cite either specific landmark studies that have changed medical practice in a particular area of pediatric medicine or that are currently debated within the academic community.

The first appendix consists of ten extended case scenarios, again with a multiple-choice question and answer format that guides the reader through the code. These cases are more complex than the opening case scenarios within each chapter and require the reader to integrate knowledge presented throughout the book. The second appendix is an in-depth list of medications cited throughout the book, all of which are commonly used in caring for acutely ill children. Included for each medication is the indication, mechanism of action, and recommended dosage.

Certainly not all of pediatric emergency medicine fits nicely into algorithms, yet caring for a critically unstable child is largely based on following specific treatment algorithms, which are presented in the final portion of this book. We hope that the algorithms in this book are compiled in such a way that they guide the reader through the thought process of making critical real-time decisions. All algorithms stem from the overview algorithm and they are all interconnected, so that the approach to every patient is uniform. The pocket card that accompanies this book summarizes the algorithms and contains other crucial information needed for the care of an acutely ill child.

Although this text was designed primarily for senior medical students and interns, we believe it will be helpful for those wishing to augment their own skills required to care for an acutely ill child. This book is intended to provide practical high yield facts and walk its readers through the many steps involved in critically thinking about and caring for acutely ill children: where to begin when approaching an unstable patient; which diagnoses to consider for common pediatric chief complaints; which labs and/or imaging to obtain; which medications to administer; when to intubate and when to defibrillate.

Kimball Prentiss, MD
Nathan Mick, MD
Brian Cummings, MD
Michael Filbin, MD

Reviewers

Josh Easter, MD
Emergency Medicine Resident
Beth Israel Deaconess Medical Center
Boston, Massachusetts

Ryan Harden
4th year medical student
University of Minnesota Medical School
Duluth, Minnesota

Lesley Motheral, MD
Pediatrics Resident
Texas Tech University Health Sciences Center
Lubbock, Texas

John Wayne
4th year medical student
University of Cincinnati College of Medicine
Cincinnati, Ohio

Brenna Yard
4th year medical student
Wake Forest University School of Medicine
Winston-Salem, North Carolina

Acknowledgments

Thanks to family and friends for their support through this effort and to future students of Pediatric Emergency Medicine. May you find your study of the field as challenging and rewarding as we have.

K.A.P.
N.W.M.
B.C.
M.R.F.

Contents

ABCs	Airway, breathing, circulation	ICI	Intracranial injury
ACLS	Advanced cardiac life support	ICP	Intracranial pressure
ACTH	Adrenocorticotropic hormone	IgE	Immunoglobulin E
ADH	Antidiuretic hormone (vasopressin)	IHPS	Infantile hypertrophic pyloric stenosi
AED	Automatic external defibrillator	IM	Intramuscular(ly)
ALTE	Apparent life-threatening event	IO	Intraosseus(ly)
AMP	Adenosine monophosphate	IV	Intravenous(ly)
AMS	Altered mental status	IVC	Inferior vena cava
AP	Anterior-posterior	IVIG	Intravenous immunoglobulin
ARDS	Acute respiratory distress syndrome	LAD	Left axis deviation
ASD	Atrial septal defect	LMA	Laryngeal mask airway
BPD	Bronchopulmonary dysplasia	LOC	Loss of consciousness
BVM	Bag-valve mask	LP	Lumbar puncture
CAH	Congenital adrenal hyperplasia	LPM	Liters per minute
CBC	Complete blood count	LVH	Left ventricular hypertrophy
CCAM	Congenital cystic adenomatoid malformation	MAS	Meconium aspiration syndrome
CCB	Calcium channel blocker	MDI	Metered dose inhaler
CCHD	Cyanotic congenital heart disease	MDMA	Methylenedioxymethamphetamine (Ecstasy)
CHD	Congenital heart disease	MRI	Magnetic resonance imaging
CMV	Cytomegalovirus	MRSA	Methicillin-resistant staph aureus
CNS	Central nervous system	MSAF	Meconium-stained amniotic fluid
CPAP	Continuous positive airway pressure	MVC	Motor vehicle crash
CPR	Cardiopulmonary resuscitation	NG(T)	Nasogastric (tube)
CSF	Cerebrospinal fluid	NPO	Non per os (nothing by mouth)
CT	Computed tomography	NS	Normal saline
CVP	Central venous pressure	PaO_2	Partial pressure of arterial oxygen
CXR	Chest x-ray	PcP	Pneumocystis carinii pneumonia
EBV	Epstein-Barr virus	PCP	Primary care physician
ECG	Electrocardiogram	PCR	Polymerase chain reaction
EEG	Electroencephalogram	PDA	Patent ductus arteriosus
EMS	Emergency Medical Services	PEA	Pulseless electrical activity
$ETCO_2$	End-tidal carbon dioxide	PEEP	Positive end-expiratory pressure
ETT	Endotracheal tube	PEF	Peak expiratory flow
FIO_2	Fraction inhaled oxygen	PGE1	Prostaglandin E1
G6PD	Glucose-6-phosphate dehydrogenase	PICU	Pediatric intensive care unit
GBS	Group B streptococcus	PPHN	Persistent pulmonary hypertension of the newborn
GCS	Glasgow coma scale		
GER	Gastroesophageal reflux	PPV	Positive pressure ventilation
GHB	Gamma-hydroxybutyrate	PS	Pyloric stenosis
H_1	Histamine receptor type 1	RAD	Right axis deviation
H_2	Histamine receptor type 2	RAD	Reactive airways disease
HEENT	Head, eyes, ears, nose, and throat	RAE	Right atrial enlargement
Hib	Hemophilus influenza B	RAST	Rapid antigen serum testing
HIV	Human immunodeficiency virus	RBC	Red blood cell
HSV	Herpes simplex virus	RDS	Respiratory distress syndrome

RSI	Rapid sequence intubation	**TPN**	Total parenteral nutrition
RSV	Respiratory syncyial virus	**TSB**	Total serum bilirubin
RVH	Right ventricular hypertrophy	**TSS**	Toxic shock syndrome
SBI	Serious bacterial illness	**TTN**	Transient tachypnea of the newborn
SE	Status epilepticus	**UA**	Urinalysis
SMA	Superior mesenteric artery	**UGI**	Upper gastrointestinal imaging (contrast study)
SnMP	Tin mesoporphyrin		
SQ/SC	Subcutaneous	**UOP**	Urine output
ST	Sinus tachycardia	**UTI**	Urinary tract infection
SVT	Supraventricular tachycardia	**V/Q**	Ventilation/perfusion
TA	Truncus arteriosus	**VBG**	Venous blood gas
TAPVR	Total anomalous pulmonary venous return	**VF**	Ventricular fibrillation
TGA	Transposition of the great arteries	**VSD**	Ventricular septal defect
TOF	Tetralogy of Fallot	**VT**	Ventricular tachycardia

Emergency Management of the Pediatric Patient

CASES, ALGORITHMS, EVIDENCE

CHAPTER 1

Basic Cardiopulmonary Resuscitation

CASE SCENARIO

An 11-month-old infant is at a restaurant with his mother and father. The child is being fed peanuts from a small cup when the parents note that he is gasping for air and turning blue. The child suddenly goes limp and you notice commotion from across the room. You arrive at the table to find a distraught mother holding an infant who is unresponsive and apneic.

1. What is the first action to take?
   a. Leave the child and activate Emergency Medical Services (EMS)
   b. Begin chest compressions at the rate of 100 per minute
   c. Perform a blind sweep of the oropharynx to remove potential foreign bodies
   d. Confirm unresponsiveness and administer two rescue breaths, and instruct the mother to call 911

The infant should immediately receive two rescue breaths through a barrier device. Unlike adult cardiac arrest, pediatric patients are more likely to have a primary respiratory cause to their arrest thus making rescue breaths crucial. If no chest rise is achieved with the initial attempts, the airway should be repositioned and the breaths reattempted. If rescue breathing is still unsuccessful, then the infant should be evaluated for potential upper airway obstruction or foreign body aspiration. You give your initial rescue breaths but no chest rise is seen. The child's airway is repositioned and the breaths are repeated unsuccessfully.

2. How would you attempt to relieve an obstruction in the infant's airway if a foreign body is suspected?
   a. Blind finger sweep of the oropharynx
   b. Abdominal thrusts
   c. Back blows
   d. More forceful rescue breaths

Relief of foreign body aspiration causing upper airway obstruction in a child less than 1 year of age is accomplished with either back blows or chest thrusts. In an older child (older than 1 year), abdominal thrusts or the Heimlich maneuver is acceptable. Abdominal thrusts should not be used in children under 1 year of age because damage to solid organs can result from overaggressive resuscitative measures. It is acceptable in the unresponsive child to open the mouth and remove a foreign body if it is visible, but blind sweeps of the oropharynx are not recommended because they may result in injury to the structures in the mouth, or may result in the foreign body being pushed further into the airway. You open the mouth and no foreign body is visible. You then perform five back blows and five chest thrusts and repeat your attempts at rescue breathing. This time, the breaths result in symmetric chest rise.

3. What is the next step in the management of this patient?
   a. Continue rescue breathing
   b. Perform more back blows and chest thrusts until the foreign body is expelled
   c. Check for a pulse and begin chest compressions if the pulse rate is less than 60 beats per minute
   d. Turn the child into the recovery position

If rescue breaths are successful and chest rise is achieved, the next step is to assess circulation and check pulses. If no pulses are present, chest compressions at the rate of 100 compressions per minute should be initiated. In a child less than 1 year of age, the preferred method of chest compression is using the two-finger compression technique if there is one rescuer, or the two-thumb-encircling-hands technique if more than one healthcare provider is present. The one-hand chest compression technique should be utilized for children 1 to 8 years of age, while children older than 8 years can receive two-handed chest compression similar to an adult. The ratio of compressions to ventilations should be 5:1 in all pediatric patients up to the age of 8 years, after which a compression to ventilation ratio of 15:2 should be used.

You feel the infant's brachial artery and detect a pulse of 110 beats per minute. After his initial two rescue breaths, his color improves and he begins to breathe spontaneously and starts to cry. You roll him onto his side and await EMS for transport to the hospital.

Answers: 1-d, 2-c, 3-c

Kids Are Different from Adults from the Start

One of the most frightening situations that a health care professional faces is that of an unresponsive, apneic, and pulseless patient. These feelings are magnified when the patient is an infant or a child, both because of the inherent psychosocial stress that accompanies the resuscitation of a pediatric patient and also because this situation is a rare event with which the rescuer is unlikely to be familiar. One of the key differences in the initial approach to the unresponsive child is when to call for help. The American Heart Association advocates a "phone first" approach to the unresponsive adult, which is designed to bring defibrillation capability to the bedside as quickly as possible. In the pediatric age group, this initial step has been modified (the so-called "phone fast" approach) to allow for 1 minute of basic life support (rescue breaths and chest compressions) before leaving the unresponsive child to activate EMS. This critical difference arises out of the different etiology of arrest in the pediatric patient. In these cases, the inciting event is much more likely to be a primary respiratory insult with subsequent cardiac deterioration rather than an initial malignant arrhythmia as with adults. There is often a "window of time" where a sick infant or child exhibits signs of respiratory compromise or shock before full cardiopulmonary arrest occurs. *This is the time to act!*

Patient Assessment

Upon arrival to the bedside of a child who is in extremis, the first priority is to determine whether the child is responsive or not. By gentle stimulation of the child, the rescuer will quickly be able to determine responsiveness. If there is any possibility of trauma, care should be taken to immobilize the cervical spine before any movement occurs. If there is only one rescuer and the child is unresponsive, 1 minute of rescue breaths and chest compressions should be done prior

Outcomes of pediatric out-of-hospital cardiac arrest

Survival rates are low after out-of-hospital cardiac arrest in pediatric patients with age, initial arrest rhythm, and etiology, all playing crucial roles. Young et al. performed a collective review of 44 studies of pediatric cardiopulmonary arrest and found that the rate of survival to hospital discharge was only 8.4% amongst 2,385 arrest patients **[Young KD et al. *Ann Emerg Med.* 1999;33:195–205]**. Unfortunately, despite aggressive education efforts by the American Heart Association and other agencies, a study of 300 pediatric arrest patients in Houston, Texas, found that only 17% of patients received bystander CPR prior to EMS arrival **[Sirbaugh PE et al. *Ann Emerg Med.* 1999;332: 174–184]**. Young et al. in a different study looked at over 600 out-of-hospital pediatric cardiac arrest patients in the Los Angeles area and found that over 50% of victims were less than 1 year of age. Neonates, aged 0 to 28 days, had the highest survival rate at 36% but the rate dropped off drastically after 29 days of life (4% survival). Survival was also found to be better in patients with a "non-trauma" cause of their illness, those whose arrest was due to respiratory illness or submersion, and in those who had a witnessed arrest or had VF or PEA as the initial rhythm **[Young KD et al. *Pediatrics.* 2004;114:157–164]**.

to leaving the patient to activate EMS (see the overview algorithm at the end of the chapter). If two or more health care providers are present, one person should be sent to call 911 immediately. The exception to these guidelines is in the case of a witnessed collapse, that is likely to be of cardiac origin (e.g., a child slumps over unresponsive while running down the court playing basketball), in which case EMS should be activated immediately in order to bring defibrillation capabilities to the patient as soon as possible.

Ventilation

If the child does not respond to verbal or gentle tactile stimulation, the rescuer should quickly but carefully look for signs of breathing and listen for breath sounds. If respirations are absent or inadequate, two rescue breaths should be given immediately. Respirations should be given via a bag-valve mask (BVM) apparatus, if available, or via a face shield or mask, and the size of the breath should be large enough to cause visible chest rise in the victim. If no chest rise is detected, the airway is repositioned and the breaths repeated. If breaths are still ineffective in achieving chest wall rise and there is no other obvious cause for the respiratory arrest, the patient should be evaluated for potential foreign body upper airway obstruction.

As previously stated, a series of five back blows or chest thrusts should be used for the treatment of foreign body aspiration in an infant less than 1 year of age. In children over the age of 1 year, abdominal thrusts can be used. Blind finger sweeps in the oropharynx should not be used in any age group.

Chest Compressions

After assessing airway and breathing, the next step is to check for signs of circulation. Palpating pulses can be difficult in the awake, healthy infant and nearly impossible in the ill child. In a newborn, pulses are most easily palpated at the base of the umbilical cord. In infants less than 1 year of age, the brachial pulse is recommended for the assessment of circulation, while the carotid should be palpated in older infants and children. Often pulses are impossible to palpate in severely ill or hypotensive children. Obviously if the child has any level of consciousness or is moving spontaneously, then cardiac output must exist. In these cases, reliance on a cardiac monitor might be necessary as to whether cardiopulmonary resuscitation (CPR) should be started. If you cannot definitively detect pulses or the pulse rate is less than 60 beats per minute with signs of poor perfusion, chest compressions should be started at the rate of 100 compressions per minute.

For a lone rescuer, in an infant less than 1 year of age, the preferred method of chest compressions is the two-finger compression technique where two fingers are placed over the lower sternum and the chest is compressed one third to half the depth of the infant's chest. If two or more health care providers are present and the victim is less than 1 year of age, the two-thumb encircling hand technique is preferred. To correctly perform this technique, the thumbs of both hands are placed on the lower sternum and the remaining fingers wrap around the ribcage and support the child's back. The sternum is then depressed one third to half the depth of the infant's chest at the rate of 100 compressions per minute. Children between the ages of 1 and 8 years receive chest compressions using the heel of one hand whether a single or multiple rescuers are present. The overlapping two-handed technique taught in advanced cardiac life support (ACLS) is utilized for children older than 8 years of age (see Table 1-1). Effective CPR, regardless of technique employed, should result in bounding femoral pulses.

Introduction to the Algorithms

The overview algorithm is presented at the end of this chapter. This is intended as an approach to any critically ill child, especially those who are unresponsive. This algorithm is actually quite similar to the overview algorithm used for adult resuscitation, given that it basically addresses airway, breathing, and circulation (ABC) and intravenous access, supplemental oxygen, and cardiac monitor (IV-O_2-monitor), which should be the first priorities in any critical situation. A key difference, as mentioned before, is the importance of initiating rescue breaths and CPR for approximately 1 minute before leaving the child to activate the EMS system. This of course applies only if there is one rescuer.

The second difference is the emphasis up front on identifying possible airway foreign body obstruction in children. While this is a concern for adults as well, it is often insidious and unsuspected in children, especially those in the toddler age group who tend to stick anything and everything into their mouths.

If the assessment of ABCs leads to intubation and CPR, basically a pulseless arrest, then obviously a source for the code must be sought rapidly. Of course CPR with

TABLE 1-1 CPR techniques for given age		
	One rescuer	Two rescuers
0–1 year	Two-finger technique	Two-thumb-encircling-hand technique
1–8 years	Heel of one hand	Heel of one hand
8 years–adult	Overlapping two-hand technique	Overlapping two-hand technique

mechanical ventilation and cardiac compressions only acts as a bridge, as an artificial means of providing oxygenation and circulation, while the underlying insult is identified and treated. In adults who collapse, the emphasis is rapid cardiac rhythm assessment and defibrillation for patients with pulseless ventricular tachycardia (VT) or fibrillation (VF). This is so much emphasized that defibrillation even precedes ABCs in the algorithms for adults.

If a child is somewhat stable in regard to airway and circulation, then the etiology of distress is obtained from the history and physical examination. There are several main categories including pulmonary, gastrointestinal, and infectious, and these are all covered later in the book. The overview algorithm emphasizes the importance of addressing ABCs and IV-O_2-monitor for any ill child, even if it is obvious that the etiology will fall into one of these categories. The point is, all sick children should be treated the same initially.

Pulseless Arrest

Similar to adults, defibrillation is also a priority in kids with pulseless VT or VF. This is, however, rare and therefore not emphasized in the overview algorithm. Children found in pulseless arrest tend to have a respiratory etiology or shock. The ensuing pulseless cardiac rhythms tend to be pulseless electrical activity (PEA) or asystole. These entities are treated similarly, as asystole is usually the end-product of prolonged PEA. Therefore, PEA and asystole are included in the same arm of the Pulseless Arrest Algorithm (See Pulseless Arrest Algorithm at the end of the Chapter). The other arm of this algorithm includes the less common VF and pulseless VT. The essential difference between the two arms is defibrillation and the consideration of antiarrhythmic agents for patients with pulseless VT/VF. Otherwise, this algorithm consists basically of continuing CPR, administering epinephrine, and looking for an underlying etiology of arrest.

The 5 Hs and 5 Ts is a way to think of possible etiologies (see Box 1-1). While the etiology of many codes may remain a mystery, it is important to rule out or treat reversible causes. If after intubation, mechanical ventilation is difficult, or if breath sounds are unequal, consider tension pneumothorax and place an 18-guage angiocatheter in the anterior chest, either unilaterally or bilaterally. A gush of air will result if this is the etiology, and a chest tube should be placed. Hypoglycemia or narcotics overdose should also be a consideration. The "coma-cocktail" consists of glucose and naloxone, and should be considered in the right patient. Hypo- or hyperthermia should be fairly obvious by history or physical exam, and they are relatively uncommon etiologies for pediatric codes. Of course, drowning and hypothermia may coincide, in which

LITERATURE REFERENCE

Automatic external defibrillation in the pediatric patient

Although the rate of "shockable" rhythms such as VF and pulseless VT is much lower in pediatric arrest than in cases of adult arrest, there are cases in which these arrest rhythms are present. When VF or pulseless VT is present, defibrillation takes precedence over all other resuscitative measures. The implementation of AEDs for first responders has increased survival in adult out-of-hospital cardiac arrest. The conundrum for pediatric arrest victims is that adult AEDs are designed to analyze adult rhythms and then deliver an "adult" dosage of electricity (usually >150 joules) if a shockable rhythm is identified. Thus, up until the year 2000, the American Heart Association recommended AEDs be limited to children (8 years of age or 25 kilograms in weight).

AED technology has improved since these recommendations were made, and many units now carry pediatric pads designed to lower the delivered dose of electricity to ~50 joules. In October 2002, the Pediatric Advanced Life Support (PALS) Task Force of the International Liaison Committee on Resuscitation changed its recommendations on AED use in children. It expanded the recommendation for the use of AEDs to the 1- to 8-year age range provided the device showed a high specificity for shockable pediatric rhythms. The evidence is currently insufficient to recommend AED use for children <1 year of age. It is important to note that the committee recommended a 1-minute period of initial CPR before the AED is used, given that a primary cardiac arrhythmia is very rare compared to other etiologies [Samson RA et al. *Pediatrics*. 2003;112:163–168].

case the most important thing to remember is that neurologic function can be restored even after prolonged periods of submersion in cold water. Therefore, CPR and rapid rewarming can be lifesaving and should be carried out aggressively.

Bicarbonate should be considered if hyperkalemia or tricyclic antidepressant overdose is possible. Both may present with a slurred wide-complex tachycardia on the monitor. Hyperkalemia may be suspected with underlying renal disease, rhabdomyolysis, or

---

Box 1-1 Etiology of PEA: 5 Hs and 5 Ts

- Hypoxia
- Hypovolemia
- Hydrogen ion (acidosis)
- Hyperkalemia/hypokalemia
- Hypothermia

- Tension pneumothorax
- Tamponade (cardiac)
- Thrombosis (coronary)
- Thrombosis (pulmonary)
- Tablets (drug overdose)

---

ingestion of potassium salt supplements. Other intravenous treatments for hyperkalemia include calcium, and insulin with glucose. If a wide-complex tachycardia narrows with the administration of bicarbonate, then a drip should be started.

KEY POINTS

- Survival rates after pediatric cardiac arrest are low and are influenced by age, the etiology of the arrest, and the initial arrest rhythm
- Unlike adult cardiac arrest where malignant arrhythmia is the most common cause, respiratory arrest is more common in pediatric patients
- The first rescuer on-scene should provide 1 minute of rescue breathing and chest compressions prior to activating EMS in pediatric patients
- The manner of providing chest compressions is different depending on the age of the child
- Automatic external defibrillator (AED) use is now recommended in children greater than 1 year of age in cases of pulseless arrest

OVERVIEW ALGORITHM FOR CHILD IN DISTRESS

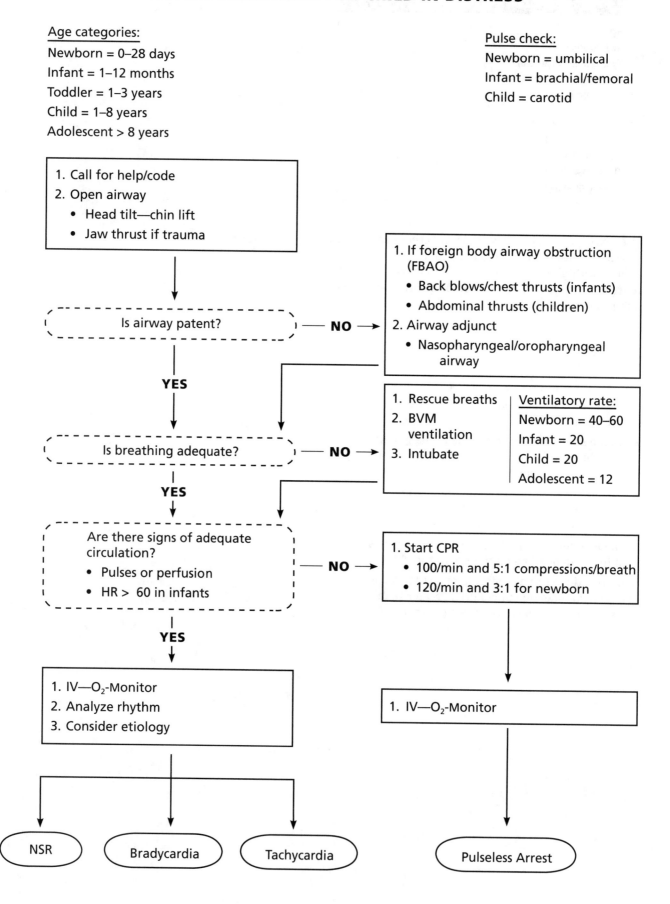

Age categories:

Newborn = 0–28 days

Infant = 1–12 months

Toddler = 1–3 years

Child = 1–8 years

Adolescent > 8 years

Pulse check:

Newborn = umbilical

Infant = brachial/femoral

Child = carotid

1. Call for help/code
2. Open airway
   - Head tilt—chin lift
   - Jaw thrust if trauma

Is airway patent? — **NO** →

1. If foreign body airway obstruction (FBAO)
   - Back blows/chest thrusts (infants)
   - Abdominal thrusts (children)
2. Airway adjunct
   - Nasopharyngeal/oropharyngeal airway

YES

Is breathing adequate? — **NO** →

1. Rescue breaths 2. BVM ventilation 3. Intubate	Ventilatory rate: Newborn = 40–60 Infant = 20 Child = 20 Adolescent = 12

YES

Are there signs of adequate circulation?
- Pulses or perfusion
- HR > 60 in infants

— **NO** →

1. Start CPR
   - 100/min and 5:1 compressions/breath
   - 120/min and 3:1 for newborn

YES

1. IV—O_2-Monitor
2. Analyze rhythm
3. Consider etiology

1. IV—O_2-Monitor

NSR   Bradycardia   Tachycardia   Pulseless Arrest

PULSELESS ARREST

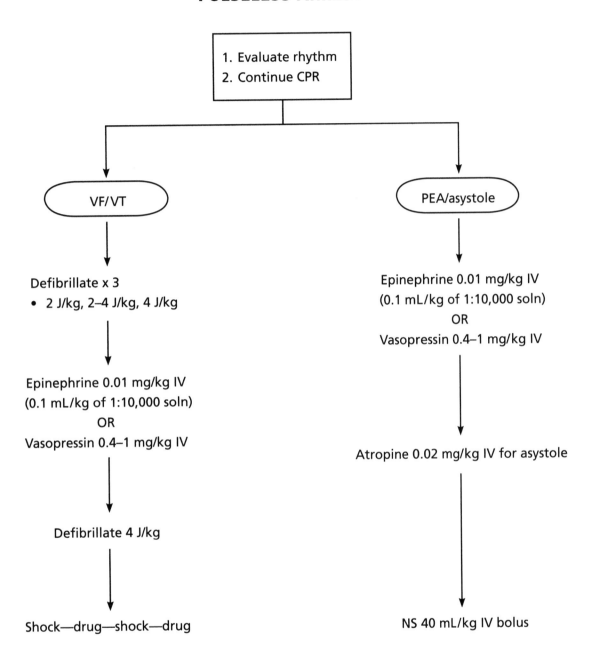

1. Evaluate rhythm
2. Continue CPR

VF/VT

Defibrillate x 3
• 2 J/kg, 2–4 J/kg, 4 J/kg

Epinephrine 0.01 mg/kg IV
(0.1 mL/kg of 1:10,000 soln)
OR
Vasopressin 0.4–1 mg/kg IV

Defibrillate 4 J/kg

Shock—drug—shock—drug

PEA/asystole

Epinephrine 0.01 mg/kg IV
(0.1 mL/kg of 1:10,000 soln)
OR
Vasopressin 0.4–1 mg/kg IV

Atropine 0.02 mg/kg IV for asystole

NS 40 mL/kg IV bolus

Consider:
1. Amiodarone 5 mg/kg IV bolus
         OR
   Lidocaine 1 mg/kg IV bolus
2. Magnesium 50 mg/kg IV (max 2g)

If hyperkalemic or TCA OD suspected:
1. Bicarbonate 1 mEq/kg IV
2. Ca chloride 20 mg/kg IV

CHAPTER 2

Airway Management

CASE SCENARIO

A 2-year-old male patient presents after falling out of a second-story window. He was found unconscious and unresponsive on a concrete slab below the window. Emergency Medical Services (EMS) arrived and found him with sonorous respirations and blood in the back of his mouth. They provided respiratory support with a bag-valve mask (BVM) and transported him to the emergency department. His vital signs include a pulse of 65, respiratory rate of 12 assisted, oxygen saturation of 100%, blood pressure of 140/85, and a temperature of 36°C.

1. What is the most appropriate next intervention?
    a. Computed tomography (CT) scan of the head
    b. Nasotracheal intubation
    c. Orotracheal intubation
    d. Hyperventilation via BVM
    e. Preparation for burr hole placement

This child is critically ill with signs of herniation manifested by hypertension and bradycardia. Although imaging and neurosurgical intervention are indicated, the most appropriate initial intervention is securing the airway via orotracheal intubation. Nasotracheal intubation would not be the appropriate airway technique because of the child's young age and the possibility of cribriform plate fracture and inadvertent intracranial passage of the tube. Preparations are made for orotracheal intubation and the nurse asks what medications you would like to use to facilitate the procedure.

2. Which of the following would be the most appropriate?
    a. Place the tube without pharmacologic agents
    b. Ketamine and succinylcholine
    c. Ketamine and rocuronium
    d. Lidocaine, atropine, fentanyl, etomidate, and rocuronium
    e. Fentanyl and midazolam

The most appropriate means to secure this child's airway is rapid sequence intubation (RSI) using lidocaine, atropine, and fentanyl, etomidate, and rocuronium. Lidocaine and fentanyl are used as pretreatment agents to blunt the rise in intracranial pressure (ICP) that comes with direct laryngoscopy. Atropine is used to mitigate the vagal surge and subsequent bradycardia that result from direct laryngoscopy. Etomidate is used as an induction agent in this case because it does not cause significant hypotension, and rocuronium is a nondepolarizing paralytic agent. Intubation without medication poses a risk of increasing the patient's ICP, which could have disastrous effects in this scenario. Ketamine is known to increase ICP and should be avoided. Fentanyl and midazolam might be appropriate agents for induction, but adding a paralytic agent will greatly increase the likelihood of successful intubation. After the medications are given, you proceed with direct laryngoscopy.

3. What tube size is appropriate for this patient?
    a. 4.0 mm cuffed
    b. 4.0 mm uncuffed
    c. 4.5 mm uncuffed
    d. 4.5 mm cuffed
    e. 5.0 mm uncuffed

One of the most difficult aspects of pediatric care is the wide range of patient sizes that must be taken into account when choosing drug doses and equipment. All medications should be delivered in a mg/kg dose and appropriate-sized equipment often relies on the utilization of various formulas. The modified Cole formula is the most widely used calculation for choosing endotracheal tube ETT size (age in years/4 + 4). For the patient in this scenario, the appropriate tube size would be a 4.5 mm uncuffed tube. Uncuffed tubes are used in patients aged 10 years or younger, due to the normal anatomic narrowing of the subglottic region. Children older than 10 years of age should have an appropriately sized cuffed ETT placed.

4. You correctly place a 4.5 mm uncuffed ETT. Which of the following would be the best method to confirm placement of the tube in the trachea?
    a. Auscultation of bilateral breath sounds
    b. Noting the presence of condensation in the tube
    c. Absence of borborygmi over the epigastrium
    d. Measurement of end-tidal $ETCO_2$ either qualitatively or quantitatively
    e. Stable oxygen saturations

The most reliable method to determine correct placement of an endotracheal tube is the measurement of $ETCO_2$ either qualitatively or quantitatively. Qualitative detectors note CO_2 with a filter that changes color from purple to yellow in the presence of CO_2. Quantitative devices may offer waveforms or an actual number. After intubation, if carbon dioxide is detected after six bagged ventilations, then the tube is in the trachea. If no CO_2 is detected, then the tube is not in the trachea. The only exception to this rule is in cases of cardiac arrest with absence of perfusion (i.e., absence of cardiac output and pulseless), where the tube may be correctly placed but no CO_2 detected because the body is not returning blood to the lungs for oxygen and carbon dioxide to be exchanged. The other methods listed are useful adjuncts but are not reliable and should not supplant measurement of $ETCO_2$ for confirmation of ETT placement. A qualitative $ETCO_2$ detector is applied to the end of the tube and good color change is noted.

5. The respiratory therapist asks at what depth you wish the tube to be taped. Which would you choose?
    a. 8 cm
    b. 10 cm
    c. 13.5 cm
    d. 15 cm
    e. 6 cm

Depth of insertion of an endotracheal tube is critically important in the management of the pediatric airway. The trachea is very short and the tip of the tube may move significantly with flexion and extension of the head. In the heat of the moment, it is very easy to advance the tube too far with resulting right mainstem intubation that can lead to atelectasis and collapse of the left lung or overexpansion of the right lung, predisposing to barotrauma. Inserting the tube to a depth equal to three times the diameter, in this case to a depth of 13.5 cm, will result in correct placement in the midtrachea. This formula holds for all infants greater than 1 month of age. For children younger than 1 month, the tube is inserted to a depth equal to 6 plus the weight in kilograms (6 + weight kg). The tube is secured at 13.5 cm and the child is taken to CT scan where a large subdural hematoma is noted, and the child is taken immediately to the operating room where the blood is evacuated.

Answers: 1-c, 2-d, 3-c, 4-d, 5-c

Anatomic Differences in the Pediatric Airway

The axiom "kids are not just little adults" never rang more true than in dealing with the airway. To start, infants and small children have a larger occiput in relation to the rest of the body, which causes flexion of the neck when the child is laying flat. Thus, effective BVM and successful intubation are more likely if a roll is placed under the shoulders to slightly extend the neck, cervical spine injury concerns notwithstanding. Children also have a relatively large tongue compared with the rest of the oropharynx, which can make visualization of the vocal cords more challenging during endotracheal intubation. The epiglottis in small children is larger and floppier than their adult counterparts and utilization of a straight laryngoscope blade (e.g., Miller or Wis-Hipple) is often called for, to elevate the epiglottis out of the way during intubation. The larynx and vocal cords are cone shaped rather than cylindrical and are more anterior than their adult counterparts. Thus, the narrowest region of the airway is actually the subglottic region and not at the cords, making uncuffed tubes more appropriate during intubation.

Remember Poiseuille's law! Airflow resistance is inversely proportional to the fourth power of the radius of a cylinder, making the smaller pediatric trachea much more susceptible to obstruction, with inflammation and edema. Croup and bacterial tracheitis that cause subglottic edema may lead to fatal upper airway obstruction with relatively small amounts of swelling. Finally, there is a tremendous range in size when dealing with the pediatric patient, from the 2 kg premature neonate to the 100 kg obese adolescent, making equipment size choice and drug dosing critically important (see Table 2-1).

TABLE 2-1 The "Formula" for pediatric airway management		
ET tube size	28 weeks gestational age	2.5 uncuffed
	28–32 weeks	3.0 uncuffed
	>32 weeks gestational age	3.5 uncuffed
	Term-adolescent	Age (years)/ 4 + 4
Tip to Lip distance	<44 weeks gestational age (<1 month)	6 + weight (kg)
	>44 weeks gestational age (>1 month)	3 × ET tube size
Oro/Nasogastric tube size		2 × ET tube size

LITERATURE REFERENCE

To cuff or not to cuff

Dictum holds that uncuffed ETTs are to be used in patients less than 10 years of age due to the risk of pressure necrosis and subglottic edema. Historically, the cuffs used in adult ETTs were high pressure, and the normal subglottic narrowing of the pediatric airway made cuffs unnecessary. Newer cuffed ETTs utilize lower pressure and may be useful in selected pediatric patients. Newth et al. prospectively studied 860 children who were intubated for prolonged periods of time. They found no significant difference in the rate of racemic epinephrine use for subglottic edema, the rate of successful extubation, and the need for tracheotomy between children intubated with cuffed versus uncuffed tubes [**Newth CJ et al. *J Pediatr.* 2004 Mar;144(3): 333–337**]. This study challenges the traditional teaching and supports the use of cuffed tubes in selected pediatric patients less than 10 years of age, such as those with asthma or acute respiratory distress syndrome (ARDS) who require higher peak inspiratory pressures.

Decision to Intubate

When dealing with a pediatric patient in a code situation, only immediate defibrillation of ventricular fibrillation or pulseless ventricular tachycardia takes precedence over airway management. The decision to intubate should be made by clinicians at the bedside and often is more difficult than the actual mechanical steps needed to correctly place an ETT.

There are four general indications for emergent airway management: failure of oxygenation, failure of ventilation, failure of airway protection, or the need for intubation due to the predicted clinical course. In the pediatric patient, failure of oxygenation may be caused by bronchiolitis, congestive heart failure, or pneumonia. Ventilatory failure is commonly encountered when dealing with end-stage status asthmaticus or children with neuromuscular disease, while patients with severe head trauma or those who are intoxicated may be unable to protect their airway and be at risk for aspiration of secretions or vomitus. There are many clinical scenarios where a patient may present with an intact airway, only to precipitously deteriorate in the emergency department, making the prediction of the clinical course of tantamount importance (see Box 2-1). Patients with angioedema, hydrocarbon ingestions, smoke inhalation, or penetrating neck injury all fit into this category.

Assessment of the Airway

Preparation for intubation should begin with an assessment of the airway, looking specifically for things that may make placing an ETT more difficult. Are there anatomic barriers such as an airway foreign body, airway infection, copious secretions, or

BOX 2-1   Needle cricothyrotomy—The last resort

In the event a child cannot be successfully intubated, a definitive airway must be established within minutes before brain-threatening hypoxia ensues. Of course the goal is to avoid such a disaster if at all possible, and RSI with a paralytic agent should only be undertaken if there is no anticipated difficulty with laryngoscopy. If difficulty is anticipated, and stability permits, an alternative plan for intubation should be devised, preferably in conjunction with a pediatric airway specialist. Most children are relatively easy to bag with a BVM apparatus if the intubation is initially unsuccessful and this should always be the first maneuver employed. It is also important to place an airway adjunct such as an oropharyngeal airway to maintain a patent airway while bagging.

Many difficult intubations are unexpected prior to starting the procedure, and there are several devices that can be used to "rescue" a difficult or failed airway. One of the most useful rescue devices is a laryngeal mask airway (LMA), which consists of a tube with a soft plastic mask-shaped end-piece that fits into the oropharynx over the larynx and vocal cords. This can be inserted quickly in an emergency and ventilations provided through the tube will allow air to flow preferentially though the vocal cords due to the shape of the mask.

A surgical airway is necessary if all else fails and the child cannot be ventilated. In adults, a cricothyrotomy is preferred because it allows quick access to the trachea. In children less than 10 years of age this is problematic because the trachea is so narrow at this point. In fact, in this age group a cricothyrotomy is virtually impossible because of bleeding and tracheal transection. In this age group a needle cricothyrotomy is the intervention of choice as a last resort. Needle cricothyrotomy is performed by introducing a 14-gauge angiocatheter through the cricothyroid membrane and attaching the adapter from a 3.0 ETT. The adapter is then attached to a standard BVM and then the child is oxygenated during transport to the operating room for a tracheotomy.

LITERATURE REFERENCE

The importance of BVM

Endotracheal intubation is the single most important skill that emergency physicians are called upon to perform. The situations that call for airway management are fraught with stress, none more so than that of the ill or injured child. Pediatric intubation is a relatively infrequent event, especially in the prehospital setting, making skill retention difficult. To address this issue, Gausche et al. assigned a total of 830 patients aged less than 12 years to either BVM (odd days) or BVM followed by endotracheal intubation (even days). This study was performed in two large, urban EMS systems in the Los Angeles area. They followed patients through hospitalization to discharge and recorded survival data and neurologic status of the study participants. They found no significant difference in the rate of survival [odds ratio, 0.82; 95% confidence interval (CI), 0.61 to 1.11], or the rate of achieving a good neurologic outcome (odds ratio, 0.87; 95% CI, 0.62 to 1.22) between the two groups **[Gausche M et al. *JAMA.* Feb 9, 2000;283(6):783–790]**. BVM is an important skill and one that is technically easier to master and maintain. The authors conclude that the addition of endotracheal intubation in the prehospital setting does not result in improved survival rate or better neurologic outcome, reinforcing the importance of proper BVM technique.

facial trauma that may distort the anatomy? Are congenital airway anomalies likely to be present, such as the short mandible associated with Pierre-Robin syndrome? The assessment of airway patency in the verbal child can be made by simply asking the child to state his or her name. Phonation requires oxygenation, sufficient ventilatory force to form words, and intact neurologic function. Crying would be the equivalent of phonation in the preverbal child. There is often a "window of opportunity" to intervene, when dealing with the child in respiratory distress before frank cyanosis, apnea, bradycardia, and death occur.

Bag-Valve Mask Technique

BVM is a potentially lifesaving technique to master. Often BVM is needed for support until definitive airway management via endotracheal intubation can occur. As with most advanced airway maneuvers, proper positioning is critical. Children have large occiputs in relation to the rest of their bodies, resulting in flexion at the neck while in the neutral position. Aligning the oral, pharyngeal, and tracheal axes by lifting the chin into the mask, make ventilation much easier. This is most easily accomplished by placing a towel or roll under the neck and shoulders in infants, and under the head in children.

There are two readily available types of ventilation systems: the self-inflating resuscitation bags and the flow-inflating (so-called anesthesia) bags. The self-inflating bags are useful in that they can provide ventilation even if no oxygen source is present (i.e., one would be delivering ambient air with an oxygen content of 21%). It is difficult to adequately provide positive end-expiratory pressure (PEEP) with the self-inflating bags and there is also less "feel" with them, making excessive tidal volumes and over-distension_a risk. The oxygen reservoir system in these bags also mandates that the bag be squeezed for flow to occur, which limits their use as an oxygen reservoir for spontaneously breathing patients. The use of flow-inflating bags has a higher learning curve, but has the advantage of being able to provide PEEP and the ability to act as an oxygen reservoir.

Rapid Sequence Intubation

Rapid sequence intubation (RSI) is the cornerstone of emergency airway management. This technique involves the simultaneous administration of a potent induction agent to render the patient unconscious, followed by a paralytic agent and subsequent endotracheal intubation without interposed BVM ventilation. RSI hinges on the premise that a patient who presents in extremis has a full stomach, making the risk of gastric distension and subsequent aspiration after assisted ventilation much higher.

TABLE 2-2 Adjuvant medications used in RSI

Agent	Rationale	Clinical applications
Lidocaine	Blunt increase in ICP	Head injury
	Prevention of bronchospasm	Asthma
Atropine	Prevention of bradycardia due to vagal surge	All children <10 years of age Older children getting >1 dose of succinylcholine
Fentanyl	Blunts sympathetic response to intubation	Head injury
Defasciculating agents: Vecuronium Rocuronium Pancuronium	Blunt increase in ICP with succinylcholine	Head injury

As with all procedures, preparation prior to intubation is critically important. Appropriately sized equipment (see Tables 2-2 and 2-3) must be readily available including BVM, ETTs, stylets, laryngoscope blades, nasogastric tubes, oxygen source, suction,

TABLE 2-3 Paralytic and induction medications used in RSI

Agent	Class	Benefits	Risks
Paralytic agents			
Succinylcholine	Depolarizing muscle relaxant	Rapid onset of paralysis, rapid recovery	Hyperkalemia, bradycardia, malignant hyperthermia, trismus
Rocuronium	Nondepolarizing muscle relaxant	Fewer side effects than succinylcholine	Prolonged paralysis (40 min) compared with succinylchoine
Induction agents			
Etomidate	Imidazole	Hemodynamically stable, cerebroprotective	Adrenal suppression with continuous infusion
Thiopental	Barbiturate	Cerebroprotective, rapid onset, brief duration of action	Hypotension
Midazolam	Benzodiazepine	Anticonvulsant properties, rapid onset	Hypotension
Ketamine	Dissociative amnestic	Increases heart rate and blood pressure, bronchodilator	Increased ICP, heart rate and blood pressure response may precipitate myocardial or cerebral ischemia
Methohexital	Barbiturate	Cerebroprotective, rapid onset, brief duration of action	Hypotension

oropharyngeal airways, and monitoring equipment (including a method to determine $ETCO_2$). Once all the equipment has been assembled, the patient should be preoxygenated with 100% inhaled oxygen for at least 5 minutes. This allows for a period of apnea without desaturation during the procedure. Children inherently have a higher basal oxygen consumption rate and smaller functional residual capacity and thus will desaturate more quickly than adults. A normal 10-kg child will desaturate below 90% in approximately 3.5 minutes of apnea, and a critically ill child with pulmonary disease will desaturate much more quickly. After preoxygenation, pretreatment medications should be administered (see Table 2-2). Lidocaine and fentanyl are given to patients at risk for increased intracranial pressure (ICP). Atropine is given to blunt the vagal surge that comes with direct laryngoscopy and to help dry secretions. In cases of increased ICP, in which succinylcholine is being used as the paralytic, a defasciculating dose (one-tenth the intubating dose) of a non-depolarizing muscle relaxant such as vecuronium, rocuronium, or pancuronium is given first to attenuate the rise in ICP.

After pretreatment medications are given, induction and paralytic agents are given simultaneously, and direct laryngoscopy and intubation are performed (see Table 2-3). Watching the tube pass through the cords, the presence of mist in the tube, bilateral breath sounds, stable oxygen saturations, and lack of borborygmi over the epigastrium are frequently used as markers of correct placement of the ETT. These signs are notoriously unreliable and should not be used as definitive proof that the tube is in the trachea. All of these findings may be present in cases of esophageal intubation, even stable oxygen saturations, as the period of preoxygenation allows for a finite period of apnea. Thankfully, measurement of $ETCO_2$ has been shown to be a reliable indicator of tracheal intubation and should be considered as the superior method for confirmation of correct tube placement. $ETCO_2$ may be measured qualitatively using a colorimetric device that changes color (usually purple to yellow) in the presence of carbon dioxide. Alternatively, quantitative monitors exist that provide a waveform and actual number in the presence of exhaled CO_2.

Postintubation Management

Once the tube position in the trachea is confirmed with $ETCO_2$ detection, ventilations with a bag-valve apparatus should be attempted. There should be little resistance to bagging unless in a severe asthmatic. High resistance should alert the possibility of a pneumothorax. The patient should be mechanically venti- lated until adequate oxygen saturation is achieved. A chest x-ray must always be obtained following intubation in order to exclude mainstem bronchus intubation and pneumothorax. The latter is an infrequent but known complication of intubation and positive-pressure ventilation.

KEY POINTS

- Children are anatomically different from adults making straight laryngoscope blades and uncuffed ETTs necessary
- Children have a higher basal rate of oxygen consumption and a lower functional residual capacity leading to a decrease in the time to desaturation with apnea
- Assessment of the airway for signs of a difficult intubation is critical prior to RSI
- RSI is the procedure of choice for emergent management of the pediatric airway
- Measurement of $ETCO_2$ is the most reliable method of confirming tube placement

CHAPTER 3

Tachyarrhythmias

CASE SCENARIO

You are just finishing your last admission of the night in room 850 when you hear "code blue room 854" over the hospital paging system. You arrive to find one nurse bagging while another does chest compressions on a 14-year-old male patient admitted the night before for myocarditis. You confirm pulselessness and note that the patient is not breathing.

1. What is your first step?
   a. Intubate the patient
   b. Establish intravenous (IV) access
   c. Grab the defibrillator and take a "quick look" with the paddles
   d. Perform a precordial thump

This is your chance to be a hero! In a pulseless arrest, the most important first step is to hunt out a shockable rhythm such as ventricular fibrillation (VF) or ventricular tachycardia (VT) and defibrillate as quickly as possible. All other actions, including airway management and IV access are secondary. A precordial thump may be indicated in a witnessed VF arrest if no defibrillator is present but that is not the case here.

2. You place gel on the patient's chest and then use the paddles for your quick look and see this rhythm (see Figure 3-1). What do you do?
   a. Continue cardiopulmonary resuscitation (CPR)
   b. Cardiovert with 0.5 J/kg
   c. Defibrillate with 4 J/kg
   d. Defibrillate with 2 J/kg

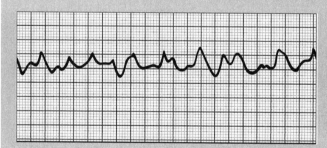

FIGURE 3-1 (*LifeART image © 2005 Lippincott Williams & Wilkins*)

This rhythm is VF and should be treated with immediate defibrillation at 2 J/kg. Cardioversion is indicated for a perfusing cardiac rhythm, such as VT with a pulse or narrow-complex tachycardia (e.g., supraventricular tachycardia [SVT]). Both pulseless VT and VF require immediate defibrillation, first with 2 J/kg.

3. You deliver a shock but the monitor does not change. What do you do next?
    a. Intubate the patient
    b. Establish IV access and administer epinephrine
    c. Continue CPR
    d. Defibrillate with 2 to 4 J/kg

If at first you don't succeed . . . Initial attempts at defibrillation should occur with three stacked shocks of progressively increasing energy. These shocks should occur in rapid succession with only a rhythm check in between. Once the paddles go on the chest for the first shock, they do not come off the chest until three shocks have been given or a perfusing rhythm is established.

4. You correctly administer three shocks (2 J/kg, 2 to 4 J/kg, and 4 J/kg) but VF persists. What next?
    a. Intubate the patient
    b. Administer epinephrine 0.1 mg/kg IV
    c. Administer epinephrine 0.01 mg/kg IV
    d. Administer vasopressin 0.4 to 1 unit/kg IV

After three shocks, the patient should be intubated and have IV access established. The next step is administration of epinephrine or vasopressin. These drugs act as arterial vasopressors causing increased peripheral vascular resistance, thus shunting blood away from peripheral tissue and to central vital organs, such as the heart and brain, which improves the likelihood of return of spontaneous circulation. The dose of epinephrine is often confusing, especially in the pressure cooker of a code situation. The correct dose of epinephrine for pulseless cardiac arrest is 0.01 mg/kg given IV or intraosseous (IO). If no IV access can be obtained, then epinephrine 0.1 mg/kg can be given down the endotracheal tube (ETT) diluted in 3 to 5 ml of normal saline.

5. You perform the appropriate interventions including IV epinephrine but the patient remains in VF. What should be your next maneuver?
    a. Immediately defibrillate at 2 J/kg
    b. Immediately defibrillate at 4 J/kg
    c. CPR for 30 to 60 seconds followed by defibrillation at 4 J/kg
    d. Amiodarone 5 mg/kg IV

After epinephrine or any other drug is given in an arrest situation, CPR should be continued for 30 to 60 seconds to allow the drug to circulate and then a shock should be given at a dose of 4 J/kg. This pattern of drug-CPR-shock should be followed for all subsequent doses. An antiarrhythmic agent, such as amiodarone, is only indicated in VF after the first three shocks, a dose of epinephrine, 30 seconds of CPR and another shock. Lidocaine is also an acceptable alternative, though its efficacy is likely to be greater in arrhythmias stemming from primary myocardial ischemia, which are rare in children. You perform CPR, shock again at 4 J/kg at which time sinus tachycardia (ST) is noted on the monitor and a pulse is felt. You breathe a big sigh of relief, arrange for transport to the intensive care unit (ICU), and finally shuffle off to grab some well-deserved sleep.

Answers: 1-c, 2-d, 3-d, 4-a, 5-c

Vital Signs Are Vital

Following the overview algorithm (Chapter 1), the initial assessment of a child in distress focuses on the airway, breathing, and circulation (ABCs). All children in extremis should be given 100% oxygen via bag-valve mask (BVM) or via an ETT. Once the airway and breathing are addressed, the next step is to determine whether a pulse is present or not. If there is no pulse, or the heart rate is less than 60 beats per minute (bpm) in a newborn or infant, start chest compressions while attaching the monitor and defibrillator to the patient. If a pulse is present, attach the monitor and defibrillator to the patient and proceed to assess the rhythm.

Assess the Rhythm

Critical to any CPR is the correct determination of the heart rhythm. The first question to ask yourself is, "Is the heart going too fast or too slow?" If the answer is

In arrest, think respiratory

Unlike adult cardiac arrest, where myocardial ischemia and/or ventricular arrhythmias are the etiology of most "codes," pediatric patients more commonly suffer respiratory arrest that leads to hypoxemia, bradycardia, and then cardiovascular collapse. Upon arriving at the bedside of a child in arrest, respiratory support should be the first priority while the defibrillator is retrieved. The only exception to this is in the case of a witnessed sudden collapse where arrhythmia is highly likely. In that case, focus on electricity first.

Box 3-1   The 4 Hs and 4 Ts of pediatric advanced life support

Pediatric Advanced Life Support (PALS) teaches that the possible causes of cardiovascular collapse in a pediatric patient can be remembered as the **4 Hs and 4 Ts.**

- **Hypoxemia**
- **Hypovolemia**
- **Hyperthermia/Hypothermia**
- **Hyperkalemia/Hypokalemia**

- **Tamponade (cardiac)**
- **Tension pneumothorax**
- **Toxins (stimulants, cardiac medications, tricyclic antidepressants)**
- **Thromboembolism**

"too fast," then the next step is to determine whether the QRS is narrow (QRS less than 0.08 seconds) or wide (greater than 0.08 seconds). Narrow-complex tachycardia in an infant or child is most likely due to ST or SVT. Wide-complex tachyarrhythmias are assumed to be VT until proven otherwise (see Figure 3-2). Common etiologies for dysrhythmias in children should be considered at this point (see Box 3-1).

Narrow-Complex Tachycardia

ST is the most common cause of a fast heart rate in children and is not considered a true "dysrhythmia." ST may be due to fever, hypovolemia, pain, anxiety, or certain toxic ingestions (e.g., sympathomimetics such as cocaine). The key to diagnosing ST is seeing P-waves, which if

present will exclude any type of tachyarrhythmia. SVT is the most common pediatric tachyarrhythmia and is characterized by a narrow QRS complex, lack of preceding P-waves, and incredibly fast heart rate, as high as 220 to 300 bpm in infants. SVT results from either a re-entrant pathway between the atria and the ventricles or within the atrioventricular (AV) node itself. Infants with SVT may present subtly with such nonspecific complaints as poor feeding, sweating during feeding, or lethargy. Older children may complain of palpitations, dizziness, chest pain presyncope. It may be difficult to distinguish ST from SVT when examining a rhythm strip. Look for P-waves and beat-to-beat variability, both characteristics of ST. Heart rates above 180 bpm are more likely to be SVT in infants and older children; whereas newborns can often have ST at rates greater than 200 bpm.

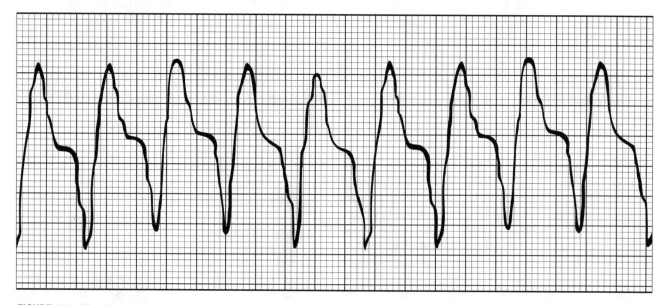

FIGURE 3-2   Ventricular tachycardia (VT). (From *LifeART image* © 2005 Lippincott Williams & Wilkins)

Box 3-2 Critical actions in the management of SVT

- Support airway and breathing
- Intubate if necessary
- If SVT is associated with poor perfusion
  - Immediate synchronized cardioversion with 0.5 to1 J/kg
  - Adenosine as an IV push may be used if IV access available and there is no delay
- If SVT is present but perfusion is adequate
  - Vagal maneuvers (e.g., Valsalva, ice to face)
  - Administer adenosine IV push, first 0.1 mg/kg, then 0.2 mg/kg if needed
  - Consider synchronized cardioversion with sedation if adenosine ineffective

---

Box 3-3 EKG characteristics of ventricular tachycardia

- Heart rate usually >120 bpm
- Rate is regular
- QRS >0.08 seconds
- QRS complex and T-waves are discordant (opposite polarity)
- P-waves and QRS complexes are dissociated (have no relation to each other)

Treatment of ST involves reversing the underlying cause and general supportive care. Box 3-2 outlines the treatment algorithm for SVT, as does the Tachycardia Algorithm at the end of the chapter. SVT with signs of poor perfusion including altered mental status, congestive heart failure, or hypotension should be treated with immediate cardioversion. Once the paddles or pads are in place on the child's chest and the monitor is turned on, deliver 0.5 to 1 J/kg of energy to cardiovert. Do not forget to hit the "sync" button. Synchronized cardioversion is indicated to avoid delivering the energy during the vulnerable repolarization period, the so-called R on T phenomenon that can precipitate VT. If at first you don't succeed, the energy can be increased to 2 J/kg. Adenosine (0.1 mg/kg IV push) is an alternative to electrical cardioversion, provided there is no delay in administration.

For SVT with adequate perfusion, vagal maneuvers, such as ice to the face, are the initial treatment modality of choice. If vagal maneuvers are unsuccessful, adenosine should be administered. The first attempt should be 0.1 mg/kg rapid IV push followed by 5 ml of normal saline to flush the drug through the line. Adenosine acts directly on the AV node, resulting in cessation of impulse conduction for 5 to 10 seconds. This will result in transient asystole until the drug wears off. This acts to "reset" the AV node and restore sinus rhythm. If this does not work the first time, then the dose should be doubled to 0.2 mg/kg. If this is still unsuccessful, then synchronized cardioversion should be performed at 0.5 to 1 J/kg. If the child remains stable and well perfused, conscious sedation should be performed before cardioversion. Cardioversion in SVT is universally successful.

Wide-Complex Tachycardia

VT as the initial arrest rhythm is exceedingly rare in a pediatric patient and most patients with VT will have underlying structural heart disease. Despite this, when presented with a patient in a wide-complex tachycardia, the safest thing is to assume it is VT and proceed accordingly (see Box 3-3). Risk factors for VT include structural heart disease, congenital prolonged QT syndrome, myocarditis, electrolyte imbalance, hypoxemia, and tricyclic antidepressant overdose.

If the wide-complex tachycardia is associated with poor perfusion yet palpable pulses, then immediate synchronized cardioversion is indicated (see Box 3-4). Once the paddles or pads are applied to the patient's chest, and the "sync" button is depressed, 0.5 to 1 J/kg of electricity is delivered. Antiarrhythmics such as amiodarone, lidocaine, and procainamide can be considered as adjunctive agents that may help convert VT (see Table 3-1). Torsades de pointes is a form of polymorphic ventricular tachycardia associated with congenital prolonged QT syndrome that is treated preferentially with IV magnesium sulfate.

Pulseless Rhythms

VF, pulseless VT, pulseless electrical activity (PEA), and asystole constitute the four pulseless rhythms and all four rhythms share a common characteristic: absence of perfusion and death or impending death. These children will be unresponsive, pulseless, likely breathless and blue. The first priority is rhythm assessment to look for a "shockable" rhythm (i.e., VT or VF). If the defibrillator is not immediately available, or while it is being

---

CLINICAL PEARL ● ● ● ● ● ● ● ● ● ● ● ● ● ● ● ● ● ●

Avoid beta-blockers and calcium-channel blockers in SVT

A notable difference in the treatment of children and adults for SVT is the avoidance of beta-blockers or calcium-channel blockers in pediatric patients, especially in infants. These agents may rapidly cause severe bradycardia and arrest in this young age group. If adenosine fails, then the next step is to arrange for cardioversion.

Box 3-4 Critical actions in the management of VT

- Support airway and breathing
- Intubate if necessary
- If a pulse is present
  - Immediate synchronized cardioversion with 0.5 to1 J/kg
  - Consider antiarrhythmics (amiodarone, procainamide, lidocaine)
- If no pulse is present
  - Proceed to pulseless algorithm
  - Attempt defibrillation up to three times if needed
  - First shock 2 J/kg
  - Second shock 2 to 4 J/kg
  - Third shock 4 J/kg
  - Epinephrine 0.01 mg/kg IV/IO or 0.1 mg/kg via ETT
  - Continue CPR for 30 to 60 seconds to allow epinephrine to circulate
  - Attempt defibrillation with 4 J/kg (may repeat in a pattern of drug-CPR-shock)

TABLE 3-1 Antiarrhythmic medications and doses

Drug	Dose
Amiodarone	5 mg/kg IV/IO
Procainamide	15 mg/kg IV/IO
Lidocaine	1 mg/kg IV/IO
Magnesium sulfate for torsades de pointes or hypomagnesemic states	25 mg/kg IV/IO

---

prepared, CPR should be started with intubation, mechanical ventilation, and chest compressions. While CPR is a temporizing action to provide assisted oxygenation and circulation, in children it may also reverse the underlying cause of the dysrhythmia (e.g., primary airway or pulmonary process resulting in hypoxia and subsequent arrhythmia). VT and VF must be identified and shocked early, as mortality increases exponentially with each untreated.

Pulseless VT/VF: Electricity Is the Key

These two rhythms are considered together because the treatment Algorithm is identical (see Pulseless Arrest Algorithm in Chapter 1). VF is characterized by chaotic, unorganized ventricular contractions (i.e., fibrillation) that result in absence of forward cardiac output. This is manifested on an ECG as fibrillatory waves without identifiable P-waves or QRS complexes (see Figure 3-3). The single biggest determinant of survival with pulseless VT/VF is time to defibrillation and therefore shocking takes precedence over airway and breathing, unlike other pediatric "code" scenarios. CPR should be immediately initiated and continued

until the defibrillator is charged and ready to deliver electricity. Defibrillate with three stacked shocks in quick succession, with energy levels of 2 J/kg, then 2 to 4 J/kg, and finally 4 J/kg. Between shocks, the paddles should remain on the chest while the rhythm is quickly reassessed. Only after the third shock should a pulse check be performed.

ABCs, IV Access, and Continued CPR

If three stacked shocks are unsuccessful in converting the patient to a perfusing rhythm, then the patient should be immediately intubated, if not already performed, and IV access obtained while CPR is ongoing. IV access in a pulseless infant or child may be incredibly difficult and if more than 30 to 60 seconds have passed or an experienced provider has tried twice, IO access should be attempted. Although central venous access should be strongly considered in the older child or adolescent in arrest, placing a central line in an infant while CPR is ongoing is prohibitively difficult and IO access should be considered the alternative of choice.

Drug-CPR-Shock

Once IV or IO access has been obtained, epinephrine should be given. Epinephrine has both inotropic and chronotropic effects on the heart and improves coronary perfusion pressure. These effects augment CPR and increase the likelihood of return of spontaneous circulation. Epinephrine should be given at a dose of 0.1 mg/kg IV/IO and can be repeated every 3 to 5 minutes during a code. Although once a mainstay of therapy for shock-resistant pulseless VT/VF, high-dose

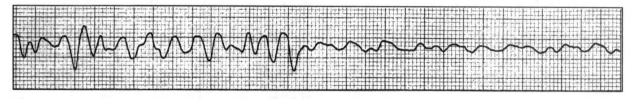

FIGURE 3-3 Ventricular fibrillation (VF). (From Senecal EL, Filbin MR. *Emergency Management of the Coding Patient: Cases, Algorithms, Evidence.* Malden, MA: Blackwell Publishing; 2005 with permission.)

LITERATURE REFERENCE

The death of high-dose epinephrine

High-dose epinephrine was long considered to be an acceptable alternative to repeated standard doses of epinephrine in persistent pulseless VT/VF arrests. To address this question, Perondi et al. performed a randomized double-blind study of standard-dose (0.01 mg/kg) and high-dose (0.1 mg/kg) epinephrine as rescue therapy after an initial failed standard dose. They studied 68 pediatric patients who were the victims of in-hospital cardiac arrest and found that survival at 24 hours was significantly lower in the children receiving high-dose epinephrine (unadjusted odds ratio for death with the high dose, 8.6; $p = 0.05$). This suggests that standard-dose epinephrine should be used for the initial and all subsequent doses [Perondi MB et al. *N Engl J Med.* Apr 22, 2004;350(17):1722–1730].

epinephrine has fallen out of favor and may actually worsen outcome. Once a dose of epinephrine is given, CPR should continue for 30 to 60 seconds to allow the drug to circulate and reach the central circulation before another shock of 4 J/kg is attempted. Vasopressin 0.4 to 1 unit/kg is a viable alternative to epinephrine, although most of the data supporting its use are extrapolated from adult studies.

Antiarrhythmics for Resistant VF/Pulseless VT

Antiarrhythmics (e.g., amiodarone or lidocaine) should be given if the arrest rhythm continues after three stacked shocks, an initial dose of epinephrine or vasopressin, 30 seconds of CPR followed by another shock. The use of amiodarone in children is extrapolated from adult data on shock-resistant VF/VT, and it should be given as a bolus

of 5 mg/kg IV. Amiodarone has been used successfully as a primary treatment of VT in children and is known to prevent recurrence of VF in adults after successful defibrillation. Lidocaine is a viable alternative, though it is most effective in arrests precipitated by myocardial ischemia, which is rare in the pediatric patient. Again, magnesium should be considered in cases of torsades de pointes or in known hypomagnesemic states.

After administration of an antiarrhythmic, CPR should continue for 30 to 60 seconds and then defibrillation should be repeated (drug-CPR-shock, drug-CPR-shock . . .). In certain circumstances, adjunctive medications such as sodium bicarbonate, calcium, insulin, and glucose can be given to specifically target the metabolic abnormalities that gave rise to the pulseless rhythm (see Table 3-2). Routine use of these medications is probably not warranted unless a high degree of suspicion exists for hyperkalemia, calcium-channel blocker, or tricyclic antidepressant overdose. After intubation, effective CPR, epinephrine, antiarrhythmics, and repeated defibrillation, the situation is grim and these additional agents can be attempted since the etiology of a code is often unclear.

Pulseless Electrical Activity: Identification of a Reversible Cause Is the Key

PEA is characterized by organized electrical activity on the monitor without a palpable pulse. Unlike pulseless VT/VF, defibrillation is unlikely to improve the situation. Instead, identifying and treating the possible reversible causes is the key. Remember the 4 Hs and 4 Ts (see Box 3-1). Hypoxemia, hypovolemia, metabolic disorders, tamponade, and tension pneumothorax are all possible causes where a directed intervention can turn the tide. Unless a cause-specific intervention is performed, PEA will degenerate into VF or asystole.

Patients with PEA should be immediately intubated, have IV access established, and be given a 20-cc/kg bolus of isotonic fluid, either normal saline or lactated Ringer's (see Box 3-5). Epinephrine is then given at a dose of 0.01 mg/kg IV/IO or 0.1 mg/kg via the ETT while chest compressions are ongoing. Epinephrine can be repeated every 3 to 5 minutes if spontaneous

TABLE 3-2 Adjunctive medications for pulseless arrest		
Drug	**Dose**	**Indication**
Sodium bicarbonate	1 mEq/kg IV/IO	Hyperkalemia, tricyclic antidepressant overdose
Calcium chloride	20 mg/kg IV/IO	Calcium-channel blocker overdose, hyperkalemia
Regular insulin	0.1 units/kg IV/IO	Hyperkalemia, consider in calcium-channel blocker overdose
Glucose	0.5 to 1 g/kg IV/IO	Hyperkalemia, consider in calcium-channel blocker overdose

---

Box 3-5 Critical actions in the management of PEA and asystole

- Begin CPR
- Intubate the patient
- Establish IV access and administer:
  - 20 cc/kg of isotonic fluid
  - Epinephrine 0.01 mg/kg IV/IO every 3 to 5 minutes
- For asystole, check more than one lead and do not miss "fine VF" that may respond to defibrillation
- Identify and treat reversible causes including tamponade and tension pneumothorax
- Adjunctive medications for hyperkalemia or tricyclic antidepressant overdose

---

circulation is not re-established after the first dose. High-dose epinephrine is not recommended.

If tension pneumothorax is a possibility (e.g., history of trauma, status post central venous catheter placement), then immediate needle decompression, followed by tube thoracostomy is indicated. Pericardiocentesis is indicated in suspected cardiac tamponade. If metabolic disorders such as hyperkalemia or toxic ingestion (e.g., tricyclic antidepressant) are suspected, then bicarbonate, calcium, insulin, and glucose may be necessary (see Table 3-2).

Asystole: Don't Miss a Shockable "Fine VF"

Asystole is the most common presenting arrest rhythm in pediatric patients and is the rhythm that is least "resuscitable." Most asystolic arrests occur in the setting of profound hypoxemia and myocardial ischemia. In children, they often begin with bradycardia, and then degenerate into an agonal wide-complex bradycardia, a precursor to asystole. Asystole is characterized by a "flat-line" on the monitor and may be confused with fine VF unless at least two leads are checked.

If a flat-line is noted on the monitor, check another lead to confirm the presence of asystole. Do not miss a shockable "fine VF" by only looking at one lead! If there is any doubt, defibrillation should be attempted, as it cannot worsen the condition of asystole. The treatment algorithm for asystole is identical to that for PEA and patients with asystole should be immediately intubated, have IV access established, and be given a 20-cc/kg bolus of isotonic fluid, either normal saline or lactated Ringer's (see Box 3-5). Epinephrine is then given at a dose of 0.01 mg/kg IV/IO or 0.1 mg/kg via the ETT while chest compressions are ongoing. Epinephrine can be repeated every 3 to 5 minutes if spontaneous circulation is not re-established after the first dose.

Putting it all together

There are many actions that must occur in parallel when dealing with tachydysrhythmias, particularly those associated with poor perfusion or lack of pulses. As the code leader your job is to identify a few critical steps and make sure that these happen in a timely fashion. Pulseless patients should be immediately defibrillated with three stacked shocks if pulseless VT/VF is present. Start CPR, intubate, ventilate, start IVs, give epinephrine, reassess, and defibrillate again if the first three shocks are ineffective. Think about potentially reversible causes and be aggressive with your treatment if one of them is likely. Do not forget about possible ingestions, especially in toddlers or adolescents with a history of depression. By having an organized mental algorithm, you can improve team functioning and outcomes.

KEY POINTS

- Tachycardia is any rate greater than 100 bpm
  - Physiologic tachycardia (ST) is a response to stressor
  - P-waves will be present
  - Tachyarrhythmia is a result of abnormal cardiac conduction
  - Unstable tachyarrhythmias require electricity regardless of etiology
  - Major differentiation is narrow-complex versus wide-complex
- Supraventricular tachycardia (SVT)
  - Fast rate (greater than 180 bpm and 200 bpm in infants)
  - No P-waves, lack of beat-to-beat variability
  - Vagal maneuver (ice to face) if stable
  - Adenosine 0.1 mg/kg, second attempt 0.2 mg/kg
  - Cardiovert if unstable or adenosine unsuccessful
  - Avoid beta-blockers and calcium-channel blockers
- Pulseless VT/VF
  - Immediate defibrillation is the key
  - Intubation, CPR, epinephrine/vasopressin are adjuncts
  - Antiarrhythmic agents are an afterthought
- PEA/Asystole
  - PEA is a precursor to asystole
  - Think 5 Hs & 5 Ts for possible reversible etiologies
  - Intubation, CPR, and epinephrine are adjuncts to correcting underlying cause
  - Do not mistake fine VF for asystole; when in doubt, shock it!

TACHYCARDIA

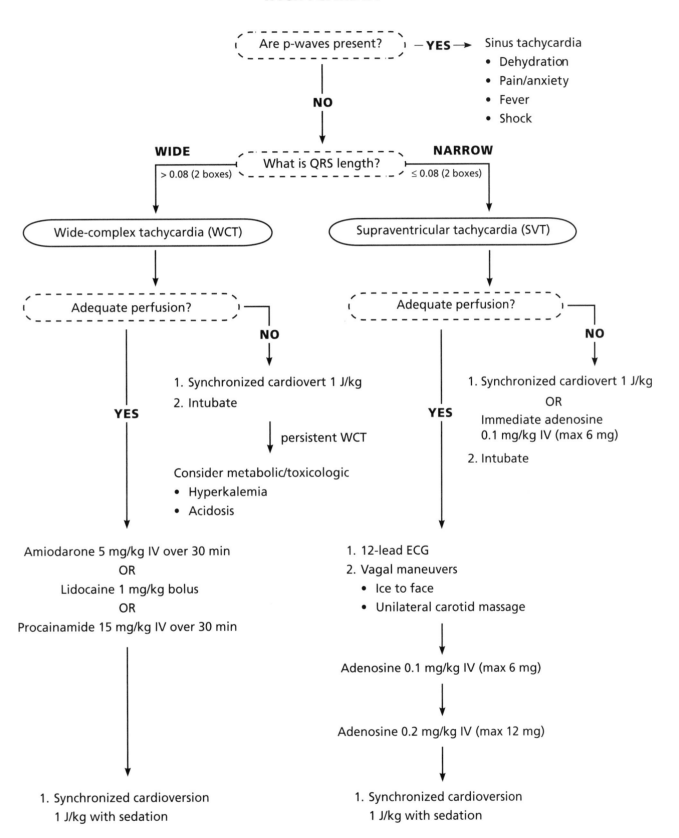

CHAPTER 4

Bradyarrhythmias

CASE SCENARIO

You are on duty in the emergency department when the triage nurse runs by on the way to the resuscitation room carrying a toddler in her arms. You follow to find a 2-year-old female patient who is unresponsive, mottled, and with agonal respirations. You feel the child's brachial artery for a pulse and document a heart rate of 55 beats per minute (bpm).

1. Which of the following is the most appropriate next action?
    a. Bag-valve mask (BVM) respirations with 100% oxygen and chest compressions
    b. Attempt intravenous (IV) access and administer epinephrine
    c. Attempt IV access and administer atropine
    d. Transcutaneous pacing

Although all of these actions are in the algorithm for pediatric bradycardia, the first steps when presented with a child in extremis are the airway, breathing, and circulation (ABCs) as outlined in the overview algorithm. Children with bradycardia and signs of poor perfusion should have their respirations assisted while preparations are made for intubation. Chest compressions are indicated for a heart rate of < 60 bpm when associated with poor perfusion.

2. You successfully intubate the patient and continue chest compressions and after 60 seconds, the child's heart rate is still in the 50s. What is your next step?
    a. Obtain IV access
    b. Obtain intraosseous (IO) access
    c. Administer epinephrine down the endotracheal tube (ETT)
    d. Administer atropine down the ETT

Peripheral IVs or an IO in the anterior tibia are the preferred means to deliver resuscitative drugs such as epinephrine and atropine. If IV or IO access has not been obtained, drugs can be delivered via the ETT. In this case, epinephrine at a dose of 0.1 mg/kg should be given in 3 to 5 mL of normal saline down the ETT while IV access is being obtained. Atropine may increase the heart rate in cases where the bradydysrhythmia is due to profound vagal stimulation or congenital heart block, but epinephrine should be considered first-line therapy. You administer epinephrine down the ETT and the heart rate increases to 90 bpm with improved perfusion. You take the opportunity to obtain further history from the mother and she reports that she found the child with her grandmother's pill box and that multiple pills were missing.

3. Which of the following medications might be the culprit in this case?
    a. Furosemide
    b. Captopril
    c. Atenolol
    d. Warfarin

This child is suffering from profound symptomatic bradycardia and the two most likely toxic ingestions that produce these effects in children are beta-blockers such as atenolol or calcium-channel blockers. You correctly surmise that the child has ingested atenolol.

4.   Which of the following are you going to administer as a specific antidote to the beta-blocker?
   a.   Insulin and glucose
   b.   Glucagon
   c.   Epinephrine
   d.   Activated charcoal

Although both epinephrine and activated charcoal both have their place in the treatment of this patient, the specific antidote to beta-blocker toxicity is glucagon. Glucagon acts to stimulate the formation of cyclic adenosine monophosphate AMP, which in turn has positive inotropic and chronotropic effects on the heart. This child should be given a loading dose of 0.15 mg/kg IV followed by an infusion of 0.05 to 0.1 mg/kg/hour. You begin the glucagon infusion and admit the child to the intensive care unit (ICU) where he recovers in 24 hours and is extubated.

Answers: 1-a, 2-c, 3-c, 4-b

DEFINITION

Bradycardia is defined as a heart rate less than 60 beats per minute in a pediatric patient and most patients will have signs of poor perfusion at these slow rates. Children are more dependent on heart rate to maintain cardiac output than older patients and bradycardia is the most common pre-arrest rhythm seen in this patient population. Although there are multiple causes of bradycardia (see Table 4-1), hypoxemia is by far the most common, making support of oxygenation and ventilation of tantamount importance. The algorithm at the end of this chapter lists the critical steps in managing pediatric bradycardia.

TABLE 4-1	Causes of pediatric bradycardia
Hypoxemia	Respiratory syncytial virus (RSV), pneumonia, near drowning, child abuse, pneumothorax, upper airway obstruction
Toxins	Beta-blocker, calcium-channel blocker, or digoxin overdose, organophosphates (cholinergic drug toxicity)
Environmental	Hypothermia
Vagal stimulation	Suctioning, endotracheal intubation
Congenital	Structural congenital heart disease, congenital heart block
Infectious/ Inflammatory	Viral myocarditis, Lyme carditis
CNS	Increased intracranial pressure

Resuscitative Measures

All children with bradycardia and signs of poor perfusion should be considered to be in a prearrest state and management should proceed quickly through the same sequence of ABCs and IV-O_2-monitor. These patients should receive 100% oxygen via BVM while preparations are made for intubation. Chest compressions should be started for a heart rate less than 60 bpm while a cause for the bradycardia is sought. Intravenous access should be obtained for the delivery of resuscitative medications and fluids. Although the venous system is the preferred site for vascular access, cannulating a vein in an infant or child in "prearrest" may be difficult. If more than 30 to 60 seconds have passed or an experienced provider has tried twice, IO access should be attempted. Once an IO needle is in place, resuscitation drugs (e.g., epinephrine, atropine, and dopamine), fluid, and blood products can be infused. Medications should be given through the ETT in an arrest scenario while IV or IO access is being obtained (see Table 4-2).

TABLE 4-2	Resuscitation drugs that may be given via the ETT	
Drug	**Dose[a]**
Lidocaine	2 to 3 mg/kg
Epinephrine	0.1 mg/kg
Atropine	0.06 mg/kg
Naloxone	0.3 mg/kg

[a]Dose given endotracheally is roughly 2 to 3 times IV dose

TREATMENT

Epinephrine

Epinephrine is the first-line therapy for patients with bradycardia and signs of poor perfusion who fail to respond to oxygenation and ventilation. Epinephrine is an endogenous catecholamine which acts to increase heart rate by stimulating the beta receptors on the heart. Epinephrine is given at a dose of 0.01 mg/kg IV or IO and may be repeated every 3 to 5 minutes as needed. If no intravenous access has been obtained, epinephrine can be given via the ETT but at a higher dose, due to decreased absorption from the pulmonary bed. The tracheal dose of epinephrine is 0.1 mg/kg and should be diluted in 3 to 5 cc of sterile saline prior to administration.

Atropine

Atropine is a vagolytic agent and should be used if excessive vagal stimuli, cholinergic drug toxicity, or primary atrioventricular (AV) block is suspected. It is given at a dose of 0.02 mg/kg (minimum 0.1 mg, maximum 0.5 mg in a child and 1 mg in an adolescent) and can be administered IV or IO. If the tracheal route is selected, the dose should be two to three times higher. Paradoxical bradycardia can occur at low doses and thus a minimum of 0.1 mg should be given.

Transcutaneous Pacing

If effective oxygenation and ventilation, epinephrine and atropine fail to increase the heart rate and improve perfusion, transcutaneous pacing can be considered. Pacing is the most effective in treating bradycardia due to underlying congenital heart disease or congenital heart block and will be ineffective for slow heart rates due to hypoxia or respiratory insufficiency.

Thinking "Outside the Box"

Although the vast majority of bradycardic arrest scenarios in the pediatric patient are caused by hypoxemia, there are several toxic ingestions that should be considered, especially in a curious toddler. Both beta-blocker and calcium-channel blocker toxicity can cause profound symptomatic bradycardia and may result from the ingestion of as little as one adult dose pill ("one pill can kill"). Although epinephrine is often useful in stimulating an increase in heart rate after these ingestions, specific antidote therapy may be needed.

Beta-blocker toxicity may be treated with high-dose glucagon infusions (loading dose of 0.15 mg/kg IV followed by continuous infusion). Glucagon acts as a chronotropic and inotropic agent independent of

LITERATURE REFERENCE

Hyperinsulinemia-euglycemia therapy for bradycardia and shock caused by calcium-channel blockade

Although standard therapy for calcium-channel blocker (CCB) overdose is IV calcium, fluids, and vasopressors such as epinephrine, dopamine, and dobutamine, researchers have found that high-dose insulin infusions can be beneficial for refractory hypotension and bradycardia. Toxicity from CCB arises from the blockade of L-type calcium channels on myocytes. In this stressed state, myocardium is unable to take up circulating glucose and inotropy and shock result. High-dose insulin infusions (with IV glucose to achieve euglycemia) have been shown to improve heart rate and peripheral vascular resistance in cases of severe CCB ingestion and should be considered for refractory bradycardia and hypotension [Boyer EW et al. *N Engl J Med.* 2001;344:1721–1722].

the beta receptors on the heart. Calcium-channel blocker overdose can be treated with parenteral formulations of calcium, though high-dose insulin and glucose infusions have also shown promise.

KEY POINTS

- Most bradyarrhythmic arrests in the pediatric population are due to hypoxemia
  – First priority is oxygenation and ventilation
- Start chest compressions if heart rate <60 bpm and poor perfusion
- Epinephrine is the first-line medication
  – For persistent symptomatic bradycardia after addressing airway and breathing
- Atropine may be used if epinephrine fails
  – Increased vagal stimuli (vomiting, intubation)
  – Cholinergic drug toxicity, also succinylcholine
- Ingestions may cause bradycardia
  – Beta-blockers, calcium-channel blockers, digoxin
  – Glucagon for beta-blocker toxicity

BRADYCARDIA

Signs of hypoperfusion? ⟶ **YES** ⟶ Intubate/CPR if symptoms severe (HR < 60)

NO

1. 12-lead ECG
2. Consider/treat underlying causes

Epinephrine 0.01 mg/kg IV (up to 3 doses)
(0.1 mL/kg of 1:10,000 soln)
OR
0.1 mg/kg ETT
(0.1 mL/kg of 1:1,000 soln)

Atropine 0.02 mg/kg IV (up to 2 doses)
(0.1–1 mg)

Epinephrine 0.1–1 mcg/kg/min
OR
Dopamine 2–20 mcg/kg/min

1. 12-lead ECG
2. Consider pacing if heart block or junctional rhythm
3. Consider/treat underlying causes

Potential Causes for Bradycardia:
1. Hypoxia/airway obstruction
   → Aggressive airway management
2. Hypothermia
   → Rewarm
3. Head injury/meningitis
4. VP shunt malfunction
5. Toxicologic ingestions
   • Digoxin
   • β-Blockers
   • Ca-channel blockers

CHAPTER 5

Sepsis

CASE SCENARIO

A 3-year-old girl presents to the emergency department (ED) with progressive lethargy. She has no history of medical problems and no allergies. She attends preschool and has no siblings. No one else is sick. Her only recent travel was apple picking at an orchard the other day. She was in her normal state of health until this afternoon when she was acting irritable. She had a fever of 103.4°F orally and her mother gave her acetaminophen. She became progressively tired and now will only stay awake for a few minutes before dosing off. In the ED, her vitals at triage include a temperature of 102.4°F axillary, heart rate of 172, blood pressure of 84/48 mm Hg, respiratory rate of 24, and pulse oximetry of 99%.

1. Which of her vital signs is the most concerning for septic shock?
   a. Temperature
   b. Respiratory rate
   c. Heart rate
   d. Blood pressure

Temperature elevation occurs through many sources and does not necessarily mean sepsis. For children, hypotension is determined by a systolic blood pressure less than 70 mmHg + (2 × age in years). Heart rate is determined by age; children 2 to 10 years of age rarely exceed 140 beats per minute (bpm). Respiratory rate is also age dependent and rarely exceeds 30 respirations per minute (rpm) in patients over 2 years of age; more important than rate are physical signs of respiratory failure.

You note that her blood pressure is appropriate for age but her heart rate is extremely elevated. Physical examination reveals a pale child sleeping and arousable for only brief moments. Head, eyes, ears, nose, and throat (HEENT) exam is unremarkable. Her heart is tachycardic without murmur, lungs are clear, and abdomen is soft and does not appear tender. Extremities are cold and capillary refill is 4 seconds. The skin has a diffuse mottled appearance to it.

2. What is the most appropriate next step?
   a. Administer a normal saline bolus of 20 cc/kg IV
   b. Immediate endotracheal intubation
   c. Administer IV antibiotics
   d. Perform a lumbar puncture

The first consideration when caring for a sick child are the ABCs: airway, breathing, and circulation. For the moment, the child is maintaining her airway and is breathing adequately, so immediate intubation is not required. It would be appropriate to administer oxygen by a nonrebreather face mask in order to optimize tissue perfusion. Circulation is the most concerning aspect of this child's initial evaluation. An IV is placed in her left antecubital fossa and a 20 cc/kg bolus of normal saline is given over 15 minutes. Given the fever and the child's poor appearance, sepsis is the primary concern and early antibiotics are crucial. A good choice here would be ceftriaxone 50 mg/kg IV. An acetaminophen suppository, 15 mg/kg, should also be given to lessen the metabolic demands of fever. After the first normal saline bolus, repeat vitals show a temperature of 101.4°F, heart rate of 168, blood pressure of 72/40, and respiratory rate of 26.

3. What is the next best step in this child's management?
   a. Repeat bolus of isotonic saline 20 cc/kg
   b. Perform endotracheal intubation

c. Start a dopamine infusion
d. Start an epinephrine infusion

The patient has now become hypotensive by age-dependent criteria. The appropriate therapy is to continue fluid boluses to monitor response. Two additional 20 cc/kg boluses are given over 5 minute intervals. Reassessment now reveals a heart rate of 152, blood pressure of 68/44, respiratory rate of 20 and capillary refill still less than 4 seconds. A fourth bolus is given as central access is attempted and a left femoral vein catheter is placed. Given lack of response to these interventions, the decision is made to intubate the child in order to remove the work of breathing and to optimize oxygenation and ventilation. A dopamine infusion is initiated and titrated up with little effect on blood pressure. The patient remains tachycardic with cool extremities.

4. What is the next step?
   a. Continue isotonic saline boluses
   b. Start an epinephrine infusion
   c. Start a norepinephrine infusion
   d. Administer hydrocortisone 1 to 2 mg/kg IV

Given the patient's evidence of cold shock, an epinephrine drip is started. The patient's main problem is perfusion and saline boluses and dopamine have failed. Epinephrine has both alpha- and beta-receptor activity; the alpha-receptors will cause peripheral vasoconstriction and raise the blood pressure while the beta-receptors will increase cardiac contractility and cardiac output. Norepinephrine is mainly a peripheral vasoconstrictor, and although it may raise blood pressure, it may worsen cardiac output.

Her heart rate increases to 162 and blood pressure increases to 84/52. Oxygen saturation remains above 98% on minimal ventilatory settings. Toxicology screen is negative. White blood cell count is elevated with multiple band forms. Serum lactate is elevated. Portable chest x-ray is negative. The patient is transferred to the intensive care unit (ICU) with the diagnosis of septic shock for further management.

Answers: 1-c, 2-a, 3-a, 4-b

DEFINITION

Sepsis is a systemic inflammatory syndrome in response to an infection that can lead to acute organ dysfunction. Septic shock occurs when the body is no longer able to maintain adequate age-appropriate blood pressure. The incidence of sepsis is greatest in premature infants and newborns, followed by children under 1 year of age, averaging about 1 in 200 patients presenting with fever. The practitioner should be highly suspicious of sepsis in any febrile infant under 28 days old. There is a steady decrease in incidence as children get older, with less than 1 in 2,000 in febrile children older than 12 months. However, there may be a slight increase in incidence in late adolescence. The mortality of childhood sepsis actually varies little with age and remains around 10%. This is far superior to adults, where mortality averages around 30%. The risk of death in children increases with increasing number of failing organs. Children with underlying chronic illness (i.e., human immunodeficiency virus (HIV), leukemia, sickle cell anemia) have a higher mortality in sepsis, and the suspicion for potential sepsis should be higher in these children.

ETIOLOGY

The causes of pediatric sepsis are diverse, age dependent, and related to underlying disease. Newborns are highly susceptible to sepsis from group B streptococcus, *Listeria*, and gram-negative rods. Children under 3 years of age have a higher incidence of bacteremia, usually from respiratory infections. The major pathogens include streptococcus, *H. influenzae*, and meningococcus. The initial site of infection may also have specific etiologies (e.g., gram-negative rods in urosepsis or skin flora from cellulitis). Patients with underlying diseases have commonly associated pathogens. Sickle cell anemia patients are at risk for infections with encapsulated organisms as well as *Salmonella*. Immunodeficient patients are at risk for any number of bacterial and fungal pathogens. Lastly, patients with central lines or external hardware in place are at risk

---

Box 5-1   Toxic shock syndrome

Toxic shock syndrome (TSS) is an acute onset illness characterized by fever >102°F, chills, vomiting, diarrhea, muscle aches, and sunburnlike rash. It can rapidly progress to hypotension and multisystem organ dysfunction. Desquamation of the skin, including the palms and soles can occur, but is often a late finding 1 to 2 weeks after onset of the illness. It is caused by the production of superantigen exotoxin by gram-positive organisms. TSS is classically caused by *Staphylococcus aureus* bacteria that produces superantigen TSS toxin-1 and enterotoxins A through E. Classically it is associated with superabsorbent tampons. TSS is divided into menstrual and nonmenstrual cases. Menstrual cases need to occur within 2 days before or after menses and the vast majority are associated with tampons. Adolescent and young women are most commonly affected, perhaps because of incorrect tampon use. Nonmenstrual cases may be associated with skin infections, postsurgical patients or postrespiratory viral infections. Patients may be more toxic appearing on examination than clinical findings suggest and may quickly decompensate and develop ARDS, disseminated intravascular coagulation (DIC), and shock. Treatment involves identification and removal of the possible source, including removal of tampons, nasal packing or any likely offending agent. Antibiotics should consist of antistaphylococcal therapy. Clindamycin has been shown to decrease toxin production and intravenous immune globulin (IVIG) may neutralize circulating toxin.

Box 5-2   Flesh-eating bacteria

Streptococcal toxic shock syndrome is caused by infection with group A streptococcus that produces pyrogenic exotoxins A, B, and C. This syndrome usually occurs with invasive soft tissue infections, such as cellulitis and necrotizing fasciitis. Association with pneumonia, sinusitis, and pharyngitis has also been reported. Patients present similarly with fever, skin findings, and hypotension. Treatment is early surgical debridement. Broad-spectrum antibiotics should be initiated pending cultures.

---

for colonization and sepsis secondary to *staphylococcus* or *streptococcus* species (see Boxes 5-1 and 5-2).

MANAGEMENT

Early recognition and treatment has a significant impact on outcome in sepsis (see Box 5-3). Initial management begins with the assessment of ABCs (see Box 5-4). Resolution of shock is the goal of resuscitation. Therapy is centered on delivery of oxygen to vital organs through aggressive fluid resuscitation, vasopressor therapy or blood products and treatment of the source through early administration of broad-spectrum antibiotics. Recent consensus statements have attempted to unify the therapeutic approach to septic patients and are applicable to pediatrics.

Airway and Breathing

Consideration for early intubation is important in pediatric sepsis. Patients may present with increased work of breathing which can lead suddenly to respiratory failure. Pediatric patients have a low functional

---

Box 5-3   Signs and symptoms of shock/sepsis

- Fever or hypothermia
- Chills
- Tachycardia
- Hyper-or hypoventilation
- Cutaneous lesions (petechiae and purpura)
- Altered mental status including confusion, agitation, and coma
- Diminished urine output
- Delayed capillary refill
- Hypotension
- Cyanosis
- Congestive heart failure
- Peripheral gangrene
- Jaundice

Box 5-4   Initial actions for patient in shock

- ABCs, IV-O_2-monitor
- Vital signs
- Foley catheter
- Laboratory studies:
  - Fingerstick glucose
  - Ionized calcium
  - Lactate
  - Complete blood count (CBC) with differential
  - Liver function tests
  - Serum electrolytes, blood urea nitrogen (BUN), and creatinine
  - Blood cultures (before antibiotics)
  - Urinalysis
  - Urine culture
  - Cerebrospinal fluid (CSF) studies and cultures (if appropriate)
- Antibiotics within 1 hour of arrival
- Aggressive fluid resuscitation
- Invasive monitoring (CVP or arterial pressure) if persistently hypotensive

---

residual capacity and may be unable to compensate for increased metabolic demands. Respiratory problems that compromise oxygenation, such as pneumonia or progressing acute respiratory distress syndrome (ARDS), may require immediate assistance. Elevated work of breathing may be assessed through

---

LITERATURE REFERENCE

Surviving Sepsis Campaign

There has been increasing recognition of the impact of sepsis on mortality. Annually over 18 million cases occur worldwide. In 2003, 11 international organizations developed management guidelines for severe sepsis and septic shock under the Surviving Sepsis Campaign. This campaign's goal is to increase recognition and treatment of sepsis. Its recommendations were published in 2004 and included considerations for pediatric patients. Many of its recommendations are incorporated in this chapter's text [Dellinger RP et al. **Surviving Sepsis Campaign guidelines for management of severe sepsis and septic shock.** *Crit Care Med.* **2004;32:858–873; also on the web www.survivingsepsis.org]**.

---

respiratory rate and subcostal, supracostal or intercostal retractions. Oxygenation may be assessed through pulse oximetry; however, tissue perfusion can be severely compromised in the face of normal pulse oximetry. Supplemental oxygen via a face mask, bag or endotracheal ventilation should be given to keep oxygen saturations at 100%. Hypoventilation, impaired mental status or lethargy may drive the decision toward intubation. Even patients without signs of impending respiratory failure or hypoxia may benefit from intubation as it lessens metabolic demand and can alleviate concerns over pulmonary edema, as aggressive fluid resuscitation should take place simultaneously. Ventilatory strategies should use minimal pressures with goal tidal volumes of 6 mL/kg

Circulation

IV access should be obtained early and in the largest possible veins. Central access should be considered as multiple intravenous therapies need to be given at once. If peripheral access is unsuccessful after two attempts, an intraosseous catheter should be placed.

Fluid Resuscitation

Aggressive volume resuscitation is the mainstay of treatment and more important than vasopressor therapy. Normal saline should be administered in boluses of 20 cc/kg as fast as possible, usually over 5 to 20 minutes Pump infusions are often not able to deliver fluids at a rapid rate; therefore, fluids should be hand-pushed in critically ill children. This can be accomplished with a three-way stopcock in-line with the pump in order to directly push fluids. Initial resuscitation for septic children usually requires 40 to 60 cc/kg; however, larger volumes may be required. An often-heard concern is that over-fluid resuscitation will lead to pulmonary edema or ARDS, and thus fluids will be limited. This is a common mistake that will expose vital organs to a longer period of hypoperfusion and lead to higher mortality in sepsis. Patients who experience respiratory difficulty or become hypoxic can be intubated. In fact, some centers intubate all patients in shock that require greater than 40 cc/kg of fluid. The most important clinical parameters to follow when titrating fluid resuscitation are general appearance of the child, mental status, blood pressure, and heart rate. Hepatomegaly can also be used in neonates and small children as a measure of fluid overload.

Vasopressor Therapy

Vasopressors are required when patients do not respond to fluid boluses. Dopamine is the first-line therapy for fluid-resistant shock in children. Dopamine acts

LITERATURE REFERENCE

Crystalloid versus colloid fluid resuscitation

Crystalloids include normal saline and lactated Ringer's solution. They are inexpensive, readily available, and excellent volume expanders. However, only about a quarter of isotonic crystalloid remains intravascular as the majority of it shifts into tissue spaces. Therefore, large amounts are needed to restore intravascular volume in hypovolemic patients. In contrast, colloid solutions remain intravascular longer and are more efficient volume expanders. Colloid solutions include 5% albumin, fresh frozen plasma, dextran, or gelatin. They carry a risk of sensitivity reactions. Meta-analysis in adult literature has shown no clinical outcome difference between the two fluid types in sepsis. There is one randomized, controlled trial comparing the two in the pediatric literature in patients with dengue fever. All children survived; however, lactated Ringer's was associated with a longer recovery time. Colloids may be better in those with a narrow pulse pressure **[Nhan NT et al. Clin Infect Dis. 2001;32:204–212]**.

LITERATURE REFERENCE

Antidiuretic hormone for refractory shock?

There has been increasing interest in the use of vasopressin (ADH) infusions in patients with catecholamine refractory shock and this is described in the adult literature. Vasopressin is a direct vasoconstrictor and has no effects on the heart. Vasopressin levels are elevated early in septic shock and then decrease towards normal over the next 24 to 48 hours. This has led to the term *relative vasopressin deficiency*. Studies in adults have used infusion rates around 0.01 to 0.04 units/min. High dose may increase afterload, resulting in decreased cardiac output, myocardial ischemia, and arrest **[Holmes CL et al. Chest. 2001;120:989–1002]**.

---

on alpha-, beta-, and dopamine receptors. Dopamine receptors relax vascular tone in renal and splanchnic beds and therefore increase blood flow to those areas. Alpha-receptors are found in the peripheral vascular bed and are responsible for vasoconstriction. Beta-receptors in the heart increase contractility (inotropy) and heart rate (chronotropy). Dopamine has complex cardiovascular effects at different doses: lowest doses affect dopamine receptors, followed by increased beta-receptor activity at intermediate doses, and predominantly alpha-receptor activity at highest doses. Therefore, dopamine can be used for different effects as it is titrated upward.

Norepinephrine or epinephrine should be added in dopamine-resistant shock. Norepinephrine is favored in warm shock (i.e., low cardiac output with low vascular resistance) for its increased alpha-receptor activity and negligible effect on heart rate. It is therefore considered a pure vasoconstrictor. Epinephrine is favored in cold shock (low cardiac output with high vascular resistance). Epinephrine acts both on beta-receptors (i.e., increases inotropy and chronotropy) as well as alpha-receptors (i.e., increases peripheral vasoconstriction). Epinephrine is therefore ideal for augmenting cardiac output as well as delivering oxygenated blood to vital organs.

Vasopressors should be titrated to effect, to goal mean arterial pressure (MAP) that maximizes circulation, oxygen delivery, and urine output. All should be used with extreme caution through peripheral veins because of the risk of extravasation and tissue necrosis; they should optimally be given via a central venous catheter. Tachyarrhythmias can be dose limiting and may require changing therapy.

Inotropic Therapy

Vasopressor therapy is usually initiated to augment peripheral vasoconstriction. As discussed earlier, it may also have potent beta-receptor effects that augment cardiac output. It can be helpful to think of augmenting cardiac output as a separate therapy in septic shock as it plays a vital role in oxygenation of tissues. Dopamine can be given as first-line inotropic support. Alternatively, dobutamine has only beta-receptor effects and will increase contractility. Unfortunately, it may also cause peripheral vasodilatation and usually is used in combination therapy. Epinephrine is the first-line vasopressor for low cardiac output, high systemic vascular-resistant shock. Phosphodiesterase inhibitors, such as milrinone or amrinone, potentiate contractility and may help children in catecholamine refractory low cardiac output shock or in patients with underlying congenital cardiac disease.

Blood Products

An often forgotten aspect in the treatment of sepsis is maintaining adequate blood hemoglobin concentration.

Box 5-5 Goal directed therapy—The significance of central venous oxygen saturation

In shock, perfusion must be restored and oxygen delivered to vital tissues. End organs can then utilize that oxygen, a process known as oxygen consumption. In children, oxygen delivery is the major determinant of oxygen consumption. Thus, oxygen delivery needs to be maximized. This is done with supplemental oxygen, blood (as hemoglobin is the main oxygen carrier), and through maximizing cardiac output, all central components to therapy of septic shock as outlined in this chapter. In addition to clinical endpoints, one can obtain a venous blood saturation from a central line to reveal oxygen consumption. Normally, about one-third of oxygen is consumed as it circulates through peripheral capillary beds, giving a central venous oxygen saturation of blood returning to the heart >70%. Peripheral oxygen extraction does not vary significantly between normal and septic states. Therefore, a decrease in the central venous oxygen saturation reflects a decrease in oxygen delivery to peripheral tissues. The latter is a function of cardiac output and hemoglobin concentration. Goal-directed therapy includes the administration of blood to maintain a hematocrit >30% followed by the initiation of dobutamine (i.e., pure beta-agonist to increase cardiac output) in order to maintain a central venous oxygen saturation >70%.

Box 5-6 Therapeutic endpoints in the treatment of shock

- Capillary refill <2 s
- Normal pulses with no difference between peripheral and central
- Warm extremities
- Urine output >1 cc/kg/h
- Normal mental status
- Decreased lactate
- Decreased base deficit
- Central venous pressure 8 to 12 mm Hg
- Mixed venous saturation >70%
- Cardiac index 3.3 to 6.0 L/min (if pulmonary artery catheter present)

This is obviously important because hemoglobin is needed to carry oxygen to end organs. It is recommended to transfuse blood if the hematocrit is less than 30% (see Box 5-5).

Early Antibiotics

Broad-spectrum antibiotics should be given intravenously immediately if sepsis is suspected. It is important to draw blood cultures as IV access is established; however, administration of antibiotics should not be delayed by inability to obtain blood cultures or for a lumbar puncture.

Glucose and Calcium

Hypoglycemia is common in sepsis, especially in infants. Young children have limited glycogen stores that may become rapidly depleted. Hypoglycemia can cause cardiac depression and neurologic damage; therefore, a fingerstick glucose level should be checked in children with altered mental status. Alternatively, adolescents may have hyperglycemia in sepsis. Administration of insulin may be necessary if the serum glucose is greater than 150 mg/dL.

In addition, critically ill and septic children often have low ionized calcium. Calcium is essential in myocardial function and low calcium can contribute to cardiac dysfunction. Hypocalcemia should be identified and treated. Replacement is usually with 10% calcium chloride 20 mg/kg (0.2 mL/kg).

Steroids

Steroids are reserved for patients with suspected or proven adrenal insufficiency. Patients with underlying hypothalamic or pituitary dysfunction, adrenal abnormalities, those on prolonged steroids for chronic illness or those who have severe septic shock with purpura are all at risk. There is no clear consensus for steroids and their role in pediatric septic shock. A random cortisol level or corticotropin (ACTH) stimulation test may make the diagnosis. Dose recommendations for methyl-prednisolone (Solu-Medrol) vary from 1 to 2 mg/kg stress dose to 50 mg/kg 24-hour infusion (Box 5-6).

KEY POINTS

- Sepsis is a common cause of pediatric mortality
  - Newborns are the most commonly affected, followed by children under 1 year of age
- Early recognition and goal-directed therapy improve survival
- ABCs guide therapy
  - Intubation should be considered early even if not in impending respiratory failure
  - Children may progress to respiratory failure quickly
  - Mechanical ventilation lessens metabolic demands

- IV access with labs should be obtained early
- Fluid resuscitation is of critical importance in pediatric resuscitation for shock
  - Large volumes may be necessary and should not be held secondary to concerns of volume overload
- Broad-spectrum antibiotics
  - Directed at most likely offending pathogen and given within 1 hour of arrival
- Central venous access indicated for persistent hypoperfusion
- Vasopressors are necessary if there has been no clinical response to multiple fluid boluses
  - Dopamine is first-line inotrope/vasopressor
  - Low dose has beta-receptor effects on the heart and higher dose has alpha-receptor effects on the periphery
  - Norepinephrine is used as a peripheral vaso-constrictor, usually in warm shock
  - Epinephrine is used for both beta and alpha effects and is indicated in low cardiac output states such as cold shock
  - Vasopressors should be given through a central line
- Hypocalcemia and hypoglycemia are common in sepsis
- Steroids are indicated in adrenal insufficiency
- Constant re-evaluation with clinical parameters should direct therapy
  - Heart rate, capillary refill, urine output, and mental status

CHAPTER 6

Neonatal Resuscitation

CASE SCENARIO

A pregnant woman of 37-weeks gestation arrives in the emergency department (ED) in active labor. She notes decreased fetal movement over the past 48 hours, for which she did not seek medical attention. Within 5 minutes of arrival to the ED, she delivers a limp and apneic baby. The baby is transferred to the warming table. You first reposition the infant's head to help open the airway. Next, you use a bulb syringe to suction the mouth and nose, all the while others are helping you to dry and stimulate the baby by flicking the soles of his feet. Blow-by supplemental oxygen is provided loosely to his face. He remains limp and apneic.

1. How long should you continue these steps until further resuscitative efforts are made?
   a. 10 seconds
   b. 30 seconds
   c. 45 seconds
   d. 60 seconds

The first 30 seconds of neonatal resuscitation should be spent clearing the airway by positioning and suctioning, drying vigorously, and providing other methods of stimulation to encourage the infant to breathe. If after 30 seconds the infant does not have spontaneous respirations, then the heart rate (HR) should be evaluated. This is best done by palpating the base of the umbilical stump or by auscultation of heart sounds.

2. You note after 30 seconds that the infant remains apneic, cyanotic, and has a HR of 50. What is your next step?
   a. Initiate chest compressions
   b. Provide positive pressure ventilation (PPV) with a bag and mask
   c. Intubate
   d. Obtain vascular access and administer epinephrine

PPV should be initiated using a bag and mask device with 100% oxygen. The mask should fit well, covering and creating a good seal around the nose and mouth only. If the mask is too large, the eyes may be damaged, or a good seal may not be achieved. You begin ventilation at a rate of 40 to 60 breaths per minute and note a gentle rise and fall of the chest indicating effective ventilation. However, after 30 seconds of this, you note that the HR has fallen to 40 and the baby remains cyanotic and limp.

3. What is your next step in his management?
   a. Initiate chest compressions in addition to PPV
   b. Continue PPV for another 30 seconds
   c. Intubate the trachea
   d. Obtain vascular access and administer epinephrine

If after 30 seconds of effective PPV, the HR remains less than 60, then chest compressions should be initiated in conjunction with coordinated PPV. You prepare for chest compressions by placing your hands around the baby's chest with your thumbs directly above the lower one-third of the sternum, between the nipple line and the xyphoid process.

4. A 2-second cycle should contain how many compressions?
   a. One
   b. Two
   c. Three
   d. Four

Chest compressions and PPV should be coordinated so that neither is administered simultaneously, since each decreases the efficacy of the other. Efforts should be coordinated so that one breath is interposed after every third compression, for a total of 30 breaths and 90 compressions per minute. Thus, in a 2-second cycle the patient should receive three compressions followed by one breath via PPV. This is a two-person job and should be coordinated well with the compressor counting out loud: "one-and-two-and-three-and-breathe-and-one-and two-and-three-and-breathe-and . . ."

You begin chest compressions coordinated with PPV and note that the chest wall is not rising with ventilation. You reposition the infant by slightly extending the neck and lifting the jaw. However, after another 30 seconds, the HR has still not increased.

5. What is your next step?
   a. Continue with PPV and chest compressions
   b. Intubate the trachea
   c. Obtain vascular access and administer epinephrine
   d. Shock with 2 J/kg (estimated birth weight 3 kg)

You now intubate the newborn by laryngoscopy using a straight blade and 3.5 uncuffed endotracheal tube (ETT) to ensure effective ventilation and then resume coordinated chest compressions with PPV, now via the ETT. Better chest movement is noted and the baby finally makes a gasp.

6. What is your next step?
   a. Administer epinephrine via the ETT
   b. Discontinue the ETT
   c. Check the HR
   d. Stop chest compressions

The fact that the baby has made a respiratory effort is indicative of a rising HR, yet you must verify that the HR has risen above 60 beats per minute (bpm) prior to any change in your resuscitation efforts. If the HR remains below 60 despite greater than 30 seconds of effective ventilation and chest compressions, then the administration of endotracheal epinephrine would be necessary. You stop chest compressions to obtain a reliable HR and note that it is 80. You continue to provide PPV at a rate of 40 to 60 breaths/min while continuing to stimulate the infant. His color improves and his HR climbs to greater than 100 bpm so you stop providing PPV and remove the tube as he is attempting to cry around it. He remains pink with a vigorous cry and you prepare to move the baby to the nursery for close observation and continued management.

Answers: 1-b, 2-b, 3-a, 4-c, 5-b, 6-c

Think Big Breath!

The most important and effective action in neonatal resuscitation is to provide adequate ventilation of the lungs with oxygen. Transition from intrauterine to extrauterine life is dependent on the ability of the neonate to breathe with a sufficient force so that oxygen enters the lungs, forcing fetal lung fluid to move out of the alveoli and into the surrounding lung tissue. The oxygen delivered with the first several breaths also causes the pulmonary arterioles to dilate, allowing blood to begin circulating through the pulmonary circuit, which has been constricted and not well utilized in utero. Therefore, blood that has previously been diverted through the ductus arteriosus now flows through the lungs, where it picks up oxygen to transport to tissues throughout the body.

Only 10% of all newborns will require assistance with this first breath at birth and only 1% of all infants will require resuscitative efforts beyond ventilation to survive. Therefore, all efforts at newborn resuscitation should begin with the airway, breathing, circulation (ABCs), paying close attention to opening and clearing the airway and getting oxygen into the baby's lungs. With adequate ventilation the HR, blood pressure, and pulmonary blood flow will typically improve without further efforts. See the Neonatal Resuscitation algorithm at the end of this chapter for an overview of the specific steps taken during neonatal resuscitation.

Airway—Open the Airway and Stimulate for 30 Seconds

The first 30 seconds of a newborn's resuscitation should focus on the airway. In a newborn, this involves positioning the baby's head in a slightly extended "sniffing" position and clearing the airway as necessary. Typically, a bulb syringe is used to clear the nares and oropharynx of amniotic fluid and secretions. Concurrently, the baby needs to be dried, warmed, and stimulated to breathe. In addition to vigorously drying the infant, the most widely accepted methods of stimulation include flicking the soles of the feet and gently rubbing along the baby's spine or extremities. At the end of this approximate 30-second period, the infant's respirations, HR, and color should be evaluated to determine the direction of resuscitation.

If the infant has good respiratory effort, a HR greater than 100 bpm, and pink central color, then routine newborn care should ensue from this point and no further resuscitation is required. If the infant has good respiratory effort and a HR greater than 100 bpm, but with central cyanosis, then 100% free-flowing oxygen should be administered so that the amount of mixing with ambient room air is limited. The best method of accomplishing this if using a flow-inflating bag is to hold the mask to the face, but with a very loose seal so that pressure does not build up. If the newborn is not breathing, or has a HR of less than 100 bpm, then resuscitation efforts continue with a focus on the patient's breathing.

Breathing—PPV for 30 Seconds

If the baby requires assistance with breathing due to either apnea or bradycardia (HR less than 100 bpm), then PPV via a bag-valve-mask (BVM) should be initiated. A secure seal between the mask and the infant's face must be achieved in order to provide the positive pressure required to inflate the lungs. For this reason an appropriately sized mask is essential. The mask should cover the mouth, nose, and tip of the chin, but

not the eyes. With effective ventilation the chest should rise and fall with each applied breath. If the chest does not move, reposition the infant's airway and try again until adequate ventilation is achieved. After 30 seconds of ventilation, the neonate should again be reevaluated based on respiratory effort, HR, and color.

If the HR is greater than 100 bpm and if there is adequate respiratory effort, then resuscitation can be halted and routine newborn care should ensue. If the HR remains between 60 and 100 bpm, then PPV should continue. If the HR is less than 60 bpm, then coordination of chest compressions and PPV should begin.

Circulation—Last in Line for a Reason

Less than 1% of newborns will require chest compressions as part of their resuscitative course. However, if the HR is less than 60 bpm after approximately 30 seconds of positioning, suctioning, stimulation, and 30 seconds of PPV, then chest compressions must begin in coordination with PPV to facilitate systemic circulation of oxygenated blood to the tissues. Two people are required to administer effective cardiopulmonary resuscitation (CPR): one to compress the chest and one to continue ventilation. Based on a limited amount of data, the thumb technique is the preferred method of providing chest compressions, but the two-finger technique is also acceptable.

To perform compressions using the thumb technique, the provider places both hands around the sternum, using the thumbs to compress the sternum and the fingers to support the spine. Remember the goal of compressions is to adequately compress the sternum against the spine, causing the intrathoracic pressure to rise and the arteries to fill. When pressure is released, the heart will then refill with blood from the venous system. The thumbs should be placed between the level of the nipple line and the xyphoid process and remain fixed on the chest in between compressions so that time is not wasted with realignment. Pressure should be applied in an anterior-posterior (AP) direction to a depth of approximately one-third the AP diameter of the chest.

The timing of a complete cycle should take 2 seconds and should consist of four events: Three compressions followed by one breath via PPV. Therefore, there should be approximately 120 events per minute: 90 compressions and 30 breaths. This cycle of three compressions followed by one breath should be continued for 30 seconds prior to reevaluation of the HR. The magic number remains 60 bpm. If the HR is above 60 bpm, chest compressions can be discontinued and PPV continued at a more rapid rate of 40 to 60 breaths per minute until the HR climbs above 100 bpm. If the HR remains below 60 bpm, then coordinated compressions and ventilation should be continued and intubation should be performed for better ventilation and delivery of epinephrine.

Epinephrine Administration

Epinephrine is indicated when the HR remains below 60 bpm despite the initial 30 seconds of stimulation, 30 seconds of PPV, and 30 seconds of coordinated chest compressions and PPV. Epinephrine should be given via the most accessible route, which in the case of the newborn is typically via an ETT. The umbilical vein is an alternative route, which offers a faster absorption rate; however, umbilical vein catheterization typically requires significantly more time than endotracheal intubation and therefore is not often the first choice for epinephrine delivery. The recommended dose of epinephrine for newborns is 0.1 to 0.3 mL/kg (typically 0.2–0.5 ml) of 1:10,000 solution. The drug should be flushed with 0.5 to 1.0 mL of normal saline, whether given by ETT or umbilical vein catheter. Following epinephrine administration via either route, chest compressions and ventilation should resume. The HR should rise within roughly 30 seconds. If this does not happen, the dose can be repeated every 3 to 5 minutes, but first adequate compressions and ventilation must be ensured. If an ETT has not yet been placed for ventilation and administration of epinephrine, then it must be placed now. And as always, the position of an ETT within the trachea must continually be confirmed if there is persistent bradycardia.

Volume Expansion

When the patient remains bradycardic despite several rounds of epinephrine in conjunction with adequate compressions and ventilation, or in circumstances where perinatal blood loss is suspected, then volume expansion to treat hypovolemia and ensuing metabolic acidosis should be considered within the first 5 to 10 minutes of resuscitation. Isotonic crystalloid solutions are recommended for treating hypovolemia and acceptable forms include normal saline, Ringer's lactate, and O-negative blood. The starting bolus should be 10 mL/kg, and a second bolus may be required. The umbilical vein is the most accessible vein in a newborn and is therefore the recommended route for fluid replacement (see Box 6-1), but peripheral venous access can also be used for fluid resuscitation, as can the intraosseous route. Rapid administration of a fluid bolus is ideal for volume expansion, but concern for intracranial hemorrhage, particularly in preterm babies, should limit the rate of bolus administration to 5 to 10 minutes.

BOX 6-1   Umbilical vein catheterization

Catheterization of the umbilical vein is indicated in newborns who require immediate access for IV fluids or emergency medications. Required materials include an umbilical artery catheterization kit, including a no. 5 French catheter for infants weighing <3.5 kg or a no. 8 French catheter for infants weighing >3.5 kg. This procedure should be performed wearing a mask, hat, and sterile gloves and gown.

1. Clean the umbilicus with antiseptic solution.
2. Tie a piece of umbilical tape around the base of the umbilical cord tightly enough to minimize blood loss, but loosely enough so that the catheter can be easily passed through the vessel.
3. Cut off the excess umbilical cord with a scalpel, leaving an approximate 1-cm stump.
4. Identify the umbilical vein. Remember, there are usually two umbilical arteries and one vein, which is larger with a thinner vessel wall.
5. Use a hemostat to grasp the end of the umbilicus to hold it upright and steady.
6. Open and dilate the vein with forceps and then insert the catheter.
7. To determine the depth of insertion, add 0.5 to 1 cm to the length of the xiphoid to the umbilicus.
8. Occasionally, the catheter can enter the portal vein. If you meet resistance while advancing the catheter, you should suspect that you have entered the portal vein and withdraw and readvance the catheter.

Bicarbonate: To Give or Not to Give?

When tissues have been deprived of oxygen, lactic acid accumulates and can reduce cardiac function even further. Lactic acid also causes the pulmonary vasculature to vasoconstrict. This physiologic response to metabolic acidosis also worsens a bad situation by further decreasing the ability of the lungs to oxygenate the blood, thus creating a vicious cycle. So then, when should the cycle be interrupted by the administration of sodium bicarbonate? This is a controversial topic in neonatal resuscitation, but currently there is insufficient evidence to recommend the routine use of bicarbonate in newborn resuscitation.

The administration of sodium bicarbonate corrects metabolic acidosis by producing CO_2 and water. It therefore can be harmful to neonates in whom effective ventilation has not been established due to the build up of CO_2. It is also very hypertonic and caustic. Therefore, it must be given via the umbilical vein instead of an ETT. Due to these potential harms, some clinicians believe that bicarbonate administration should be reserved for patients who have received

TABLE 6-1 Know your meds!

Medication	Recommended concentration	Recommended route	Recommended dose	Recommended rate of administration
Epinephrine	1:10,000	ETT or IV	0.1 to 0.3 mL/kg of 1:10,000	Rapidly!
Sodium bicarbonate	4.2% solution	Umbilical vein	2 mEq/kg or 4 mL/kg of 4.2% solution	Slowly! 1 mEq/kg/min
Naloxone hydrochloride	1.0 mg/mL	ETT or IV; IM or SC acceptable	0.1 mg/kg	Rapidly!
Normal saline (NS)	0.9% NS	Umbilical vein	10 mL/kg	5 to 10 min

proper fluid resuscitation and who continue to have a confirmed severe metabolic acidosis with normal CO_2 levels (see Table 6-1).

SPECIAL CONSIDERATIONS

Muddy Waters: Meconium-Stained Amniotic Fluid

Meconium complicates approximately 12% of all deliveries. The exact mechanism for in utero passage of meconium is unknown, but it is believed to be indicative of fetal distress (i.e., hypoxia, acidemia or infection) and, therefore, any infant born through meconium should be considered high-risk. If the amniotic fluid contains any meconium, thick or thin, then several guidelines should be followed in an effort to decrease the risk of meconium aspiration syndrome. The first intervention should be performed by the delivery physician, after delivery of the head but before delivery of the shoulders. This involves thorough suctioning of the nose, mouth, and pharynx with either a bulb syringe or large-bore suction catheter prior to the delivery of the shoulders and body. This is done to prevent further aspiration of meconium as the chest wall is allowed to expand and air is drawn into the lungs.

Any subsequent intervention is based on the level of vigor at birth. If the infant has absent or depressed respirations, HR less than 100 bpm, or decreased muscle tone, then immediate suctioning of the trachea using direct laryngoscopy is indicated to remove any meconium from the hypopharynx. Warmth should be provided, but drying and stimulation should generally be delayed in such infants until the completion of tracheal suctioning. If the infant is vigorous with a strong cry and HR greater than 100, then routine newborn care is indicated. Meconium-stained infants who are initially vigorous yet who subsequently go on to develop apnea or respiratory distress should receive tracheal suctioning prior to PPV.

LITERATURE REFERENCE

Meconium: Intrapartum oropharyngeal suctioning is key!

In 2000, Wiswell et al. confirmed the effectiveness of intrapartum suctioning in a randomized trial that evaluated delivery-room management of the vigorous infant born through meconium-stained amniotic fluid (MSAF). Two thousand ninety-four neonates were studied. Infants were randomized to receive intubation and tracheal suctioning in the delivery room (traditionally considered standard of care in the setting of MSAF) or they were managed expectantly and treated only if they developed symptoms of respiratory distress. One hundred forty-nine (7.1%) of enrolled infants subsequently developed respiratory distress, 62 (3%) of whom were diagnosed with meconium aspiration syndrome (MAS) and 87 (4.2%) of whom were diagnosed with other respiratory disorders (including transient tachypnea, delayed transition from fetal circulation, sepsis, and persistent pulmonary hypertension of the newborn). There was no significant difference in the rate of MAS in those intubated (3.2%) and those not intubated (2.7%). In addition, there was no difference between the groups in subanalyses that adjusted for the thickness of the meconium in the amniotic fluid. The study found a difference in the rate of MAS in those who did not receive intrapartum oropharyngeal suction before delivery of the shoulders compared with those who received suctioning (8.5% vs 2.7%) **[Wiswell TE et al. *Pediatrics.* 2000; 105:1–7]**.

In addition, there is an increased risk for pneumothorax in this setting, and therefore one should have a low threshold for evaluation and treatment of this potential complication.

Don't Miss a Pneumothorax!

The development of a pneumothorax should be ruled out in any newborn with sudden onset of respiratory distress. On physical examination, breath sounds may be diminished on the affected side, although this finding may be difficult to appreciate. A chest x-ray provides a definitive diagnosis; however, obtaining a chest film may cause significant delay. Transillumination is a useful technique to diagnose a pneumothorax immediately by revealing hyperlucency on the affected side. The unaffected side will not light up as intensely. Rapid decompression of a symptomatic pneumothorax is best achieved by inserting an intravenous (IV) catheter in the second intercostal space along the mid-clavicular line, removing the stylet, and aspirating while advancing the catheter. Subsequent chest tube placement can take place under sterile conditions if a more permanent evacuation device is required.

Know Your Narcan "'No-No's"

Naloxone hydrochloride (Narcan) provides narcotic antagonism. It should be used in a newborn with respiratory depression, whose mother received narcotics within 4 hours of delivery. It should not, however, be used in any infant whose mother is suspected of narcotics abuse because it may precipitate abrupt and severe withdrawal signs, including seizures, in such infants. The recommended dose is 0.1 mg/kg given intravenously, endotracheally, or even intramuscularly (IM) in patients with adequate circulation (see Table 6-1).

KEY POINTS

- Hypoxia is almost always present in any newborn requiring resuscitation
  - Administration of 100% oxygen is indicated
  - Determine the need for further resuscitation
- Indications for PPV
  - Apnea or gasping respirations
  - HR < 100 bpm
  - Persistent central cyanosis despite 100% oxygen
- PPV should be delivered at a rate of 40 to 60 per minute for 30 seconds
- Chest compressions (CPR) should be administered for HR < 60 bpm despite adequate assisted ventilation for 30 seconds
  - Two-thumb method of chest compression is preferred
  - Depth of compression one-third the AP diameter of the chest
  - Rate of 90 compressions in 60 seconds coordinated with 30 breaths
- Epinephrine should be administered if the HR remains < 60 bpm after a minimum of 30 seconds of CPR
  - Dose of 0.01 to 0.03 mg/kg (0.1–0.3 mL/kg of 1:10,000 solution)
- Emergency volume expansion should be considered
  - Isotonic crystalloid solution or O-negative blood
  - Dose of 10 mL/kg given over 5 to 10 minutes
- Umbilical vein catheterization is the access of choice for newborns
  - Intraosseous or peripheral access can serve as an alternative route
- Infants delivered through meconium require intubation with tracheal suctioning if not "vigorous" at birth defined by:
  - Strong respiratory efforts
  - Good muscle tone
  - HR > 100 bpm
- Never give Narcan to an infant whose mother is suspected of narcotics abuse
  - May precipitate severe withdrawal or seizures
- Suspect a pneumothorax if a newborn acutely develops respiratory distress
  - Particularly in infants born through meconium

NEONATAL RESUSCITATION

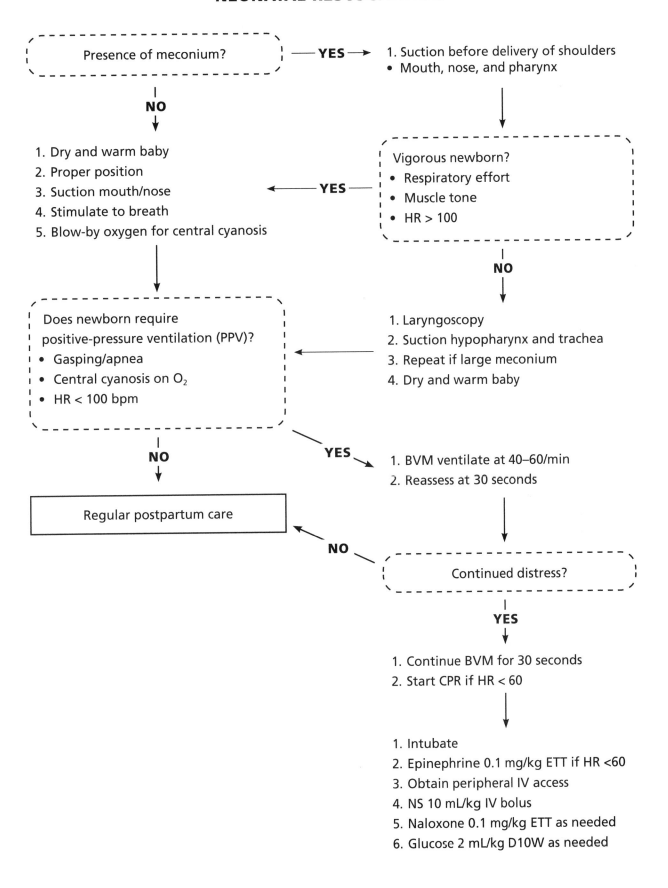

Presence of meconium?

— YES →

1. Suction before delivery of shoulders
   - Mouth, nose, and pharynx

NO

1. Dry and warm baby
2. Proper position
3. Suction mouth/nose
4. Stimulate to breath
5. Blow-by oxygen for central cyanosis

Vigorous newborn?
- Respiratory effort
- Muscle tone
- HR > 100

← YES —

NO

Does newborn require
positive-pressure ventilation (PPV)?
- Gasping/apnea
- Central cyanosis on O_2
- HR < 100 bpm

1. Laryngoscopy
2. Suction hypopharynx and trachea
3. Repeat if large meconium
4. Dry and warm baby

NO

YES

1. BVM ventilate at 40–60/min
2. Reassess at 30 seconds

Regular postpartum care

NO

Continued distress?

YES

1. Continue BVM for 30 seconds
2. Start CPR if HR < 60

1. Intubate
2. Epinephrine 0.1 mg/kg ETT if HR <60
3. Obtain peripheral IV access
4. NS 10 mL/kg IV bolus
5. Naloxone 0.1 mg/kg ETT as needed
6. Glucose 2 mL/kg D10W as needed

CHAPTER 7

Fever: 0–3 Months

CASE SCENARIO

A 4-day-old female infant presents to the ED for evaluation of fever. According to the mother, the child was seen in her pediatrician's office today for a routine visit after being discharged from the newborn nursery 2 days ago and was noted to have a fever to 38.6°C. The mother reports that the child is the term product of a normal spontaneous vaginal delivery and had no perinatal problems. She is being exclusively breast-fed and has had decreased appetite and a decrease in the number of wet diapers over the past 24 hours. The infant's vital signs include a heart rate of 180, a respiratory rate of 30, and a blood pressure of 60/40. The child is noted to be irritable and to have a bulging fontanel.

1. Which of the following organisms is most likely responsible for this child's illness?
    a. Group B streptococcus
    b. *Listeria monocytogenes*
    c. *Streptococcus pneumoniae*
    d. *Haemophilus influenzae*
    e. *Escherichia coli*

This infant has signs and symptoms of meningitis including irritability, tachycardia, and hypotension. Any of the above organisms could potentially be the culprit, although group B streptococcus is the most common offender at this early age. Group B streptococcus, *Listeria*, and *E. coli* are important pathogens in this age group and are transmitted vertically from the birth canal. *S. pneumoniae* and *H. influenzae* can cause meningitis in any age group, but the incidence of invasive disease has decreased in older children who are completely immunized. The child is placed on a monitor.

2. Which of the following should be obtained as part of the ED evaluation of this neonate?
    a. Cerebrospinal fluid (CSF) for analysis and culture
    b. Complete blood count (CBC) and blood culture
    c. Urinalysis (UA) and urine culture
    d. CBC, blood culture, UA and urine culture, and CSF for analysis and culture

The child in this vignette is at particular risk for meningitis and disseminated bacteremia due to her age and the fact that she is not immunized against *H. influenzae* (HIB vaccine) and *S. pneumoniae* (pneumococcal heptavalent conjugate vaccine, Prevnar). In this age group, classic signs of meningitis including altered mental status, neck stiffness, and headache are often not present and fever may be the only sign of bacterial infection. Thus, infants less than 28 days with a fever greater than 38°C should have blood, urine, and CSF cultures obtained and receive empiric parenteral antibiotics.

3. What is an appropriate initial antibiotic regimen for this infant?
    a. Ceftriaxone 50 mg/kg IV
    b. Ceftriaxone 100 mg/kg IV
    c. Ampicillin IV and gentamicin IV and cafotaxine
    d. Cefotaxime IV and metronidazole IV

An appropriate antibiotic regimen for this infant would cover the most likely causative organisms in this age group (group B streptococci, *L. monocytogenes, S. pneumonia*, and *H. influenzae*). Although ceftriaxone is widely used for initial empiric coverage in older children, it is ineffective against *L. monocytogenes* and is relatively contraindicated in the neonatal period because it displaces bilirubin from its protein binding sites. Thus, in the infant who is already jaundiced, it can theoretically worsen hyperbilirubinemia and precipitate acute bilirubin encephalopathy. Ampicillin provides excellent coverage against *L. monocytogenes* with coverage of group B strep as well cefotaxime and gentamicin have excellent gram-negative coverage with the additional benefit that cefotaxime readily crosses the blood-brain barrier and in combination both have synergistic effects against gram-positive organisms. The child should then be admitted to the hospital until blood, urine, and CSF cultures are negative.

Answers: 1-a, 2-d, 3-c

APPROACH TO FEVER IN INFANTS

Fever is one of the most common chief complaints of pediatric patients presenting to the ED and can have a myriad of causes which range from the benign to the immediately life threatening (see Box 7-1). Although it is important to consider other entities in the differential of the child who presents with an elevated temperature, the most common causes of fever are still infectious. The evaluation of the febrile infant depends on multiple factors including the age of the patient, birth history and complications, whether the child is "toxic" appearing, exposures, immune status, and the presence of an infectious source identified on examination. In the 0 to 3 month age group, a "significant" fever is defined as a core temperature greater than 38°C (100.4°F).

Generally, all febrile children should be assessed for signs of systemic infection and sepsis. Signs and symptoms of sepsis include tachycardia, hypotension, tachypnea, poor perfusion, lethargy, and altered mental status. All ill-appearing children should be placed on a monitor, given supplemental oxygen, and have intravenous access obtained. If possible, CSF, blood, and urine cultures should be obtained prior to the administration of broad-spectrum empiric antibiotics. Tachypnea and respiratory distress may herald an infectious pulmonary process or be caused by the increased metabolic demands of systemic illness. Severe respiratory distress may warrant definitive airway management via endotracheal intubation. Hypotension and signs of shock including poor perfusion, lethargy, altered mental status, and decreased urine output should be treated with 20 cc/kg boluses of isotonic fluids (Ringer's lactate or normal saline). Hypotension unresponsive to three 20 cc/kg boluses of fluid may be treated with vasopressor agents such as dopamine or norepinephrine.

Diagnostic evaluation of infants less than 3 months of age with fever should focus on excluding serious bacterial illness (SBI), which includes

BOX 7-1 Etiology of fever in children	
Infectious	**Malignancy**
Viral	Leukemia
Influenza	Lymphoma
Respiratory syncytial virus	Neuroblastoma
Parainfluenza	Ewing sarcoma
Adenovirus	Wilms tumor
Rhinovirus	
Cytomegalovirus (CMV)	**Injury**
Epstein-Barr virus (EBV)	Burns
Coxsackie	Trauma
Bacterial	Tissue Infarction
S. pneumonia	Pulmonary embolism
Group A streptococcus	
Staphylococcus aureus	**Drugs**
Salmonella	Cocaine
H. influenzae	Interferon
Moraxella	Amphotericin
Mycoplasma	
Parasitic	**Endocrine**
Giardia	Thyrotoxicosis
Amebiasis	Pheochromocytoma
Malaria	
Fungal	**Metabolic/Genetic**
Spirochetes	Gout
Lyme disease	Uremia
Syphilis	Familial
	Mediterranean fever
Rheumatologic/Inflammatory	Vaccines
Inflammatory bowel disease	
Crohn disease and	Blood infusion
ulcerative colitis	
Kawasaki disease	
Lupus	Factitious
Juvenile rheumatoid arthritis	
Rheumatic fever	
Dermatomyositis	
Sarcoidosis	

LITERATURE REFERENCE

Prevalence of SBI in febrile infants less than 3 months of age

One may ask why we take fever so seriously in infants less than 3 months of age. While many of these infants may "look well" and one may be tempted to just send them home with Tylenol (acetaminophen), the data show that these children have a significant incidence of SBI that in the worst case may progress to sepsis, meningitis, and death. A review of 18 studies with more than 6,300 patients by Slater et al. revealed a cumulative SBI rate of 9% in febrile infants less than 3 months of age [Slater M et al. *Emerg Med Clin North Am.* 1999;17:97–126].

BOX 7-2   Common bacterial causes of illness by age

0 to 28 days
Group B streptococcus
Listeria monocytogenes
Streptococcus pneumoniae
Haemophilus influenzae B
Escherichia coli
HSV*

1 to 3 months
Group B streptococcus
Staphylococcus aureus
Streptococcus pneumoniae
Haemophilus influenzae B
Neisseria meningitidis

*Viral illness that may cause neonatal sepsis and meningoencephalitis

meningitis, pneumonia, urinary tract infection (UTI), bacteremia, bacterial enteritis, and other skin, bone, and soft-tissue infections. Rates of SBI in febrile infants less than 3 months of age range from 6% to 10%, and unfortunately few of these have overt clinical evidence of an infectious source on physical examination. Much research has been conducted searching for the perfect strategy for the management of young febrile infants. Significant controversy still exists and multiple strategies reported and tested in the literature, differ in the age of inclusion, the definition of significant fever, and the appropriate diagnostic evaluation. The algorithm at the end of this chapter summarizes the fever workup for children from 0 to 3 months of age, and it represents the more conservative of the several approaches used in practice.

NEONATES (0–28 DAYS OLD)

Neonates are at increased risk for perinatal as well as community-acquired infections. Box 7-2 shows common perinatal organisms. Neonates do not localize infection well due to the immaturity of their immune systems which places them at risk for serious bacterial infection and spread of infection from relatively "minor" sites (e.g., cellulitis or otitis media). Very little controversy exists in the management of these infants. They all require a complete sepsis evaluation including CBC with differential and blood culture, UA and urine culture, and CSF cell count and culture.

All febrile children less than 28 days old require admission to the hospital for parenteral antibiotics, regardless of how well they look.

The classic treatment for fever in this age group consists of gentamicin and ampicillin. Gentamicin covers gram-negative organisms and group B streptococcus (GBS). Ampicillin covers *Listeria* and is synergistic with gentamicin against GBS. Some providers will use cefotaxime instead of gentamicin because it has good CSF penetration and fewer side effects. Ceftriaxone is avoided in this age because it displaces bilirubin from albumin, increasing the risk of jaundice and kernicterus. In addition, acyclovir is often added to cover against possible herpes simplex virus (HSV) infection. Maternal history of HSV or high number of red cells in the CSF may suggest herpes encephalitis; however, most children with HSV have no maternal history and a normal number of red blood cells in the CSF. Detection of HSV via polymerase chain reaction (PCR) of the CSF is sensitive and relatively rapid, with results usually available within 24 hours. Most bacterial cultures will be positive within 36 to 48 hours.

INFANTS (1–3 MONTHS OLD)

While infants from 1 to 3 months of age are less likely to have perinatal-acquired infection, they still have a similar risk for SBI. Infants up to 6 weeks are at risk for late-onset GBS or *Listeria* sepsis. After 6 weeks, infants are more at risk for community-acquired pathogens such as streptococcus and *H. influenzae*. Multiple strategies have been developed for the evaluation of the febrile infant 1 to 3 months of age, and two of the more commonly used strategies are presented here along with the evidence to back them up.

Baskin et al. evaluated over 500 febrile infants between 28 and 89 days of age and divided them into low-risk and high-risk groups. All children received a CBC with differential, blood culture, UA and culture, and CSF analysis and culture. A child was considered high risk if any of the following was met:

1. Presence of bacterial infection on physical examination (e.g., otitis media, cellulitis, osteomyelitis)

2. CSF white blood cell (WBC) count >10 cells/mm^3

3. UA with >10 WBCs/hpf

4. WBC count >20,000

5. Infiltrate on chest radiograph, if obtained

High-risk patients were admitted for IV antibiotics. If none of these criteria were met (i.e., low risk) the patient was given ceftriaxone 50 mg/kg intramuscularly prior to discharge and had follow-up the next day either in the ED or with their primary care physician. Approximately two-thirds of the febrile infants qualified as low risk and were discharged home. Nine of the "low-risk" patients were found to have bacteremia, all of whom were subsequently admitted and did well. By utilizing these criteria, the authors were able to discharge two-thirds of febrile infants from the ED but they concluded that "low-risk" does not equate to "no-risk" making empiric antibiotics necessary [Baskin MN et al. *J Pediatr.* 1992;120:22–27].

Investigators in Philadelphia subsequently developed a set of criteria designed to identify low-risk infants aged 29 to 60 days who could be safely managed as outpatients without antibiotics. They examined 747 well-appearing infants with fever <38.2°C and no focus of infection on examination. All enrolled patients had a CBC with differential, blood culture, UA and culture, and CSF analysis and culture. High risk was defined as (1) WBC > 15,000/mm^3, (2) UA with greater than 10 WBCs/hpf or bacteriuria, (3) CSF with greater than 8 WBCs or bacteria seen on gram stain, (4) Positive findings on chest radiograph or stool studies, if obtained. All high-risk patients were admitted for parenteral antibiotics. Low-risk patients were randomized to one of two groups: (1) Admission to the hospital without antibiotics or (2) Discharged home without antibiotics. Approximately 61% of patients were high risk and were admitted to the hospital; 19% were low risk and admitted, and 20% were low risk and discharged. The "Philadelphia criteria" were found to have a negative predictive value of 99.7% for identifying SBI (i.e., if none of the above criteria were

met, the infant had extremely small chance of SBI). The authors concluded that it was possible to identify a group of febrile infants 1 to 2 months of age who could safely be discharged home without antibiotic therapy [Baker MD et al. *N Engl J Med.* 1993;329:1437–1441]. Regardless, it is important to remember that both strategies involve a full sepsis workup for all febrile infants less than 60 days of age.

Less Stringent Criteria for 61 to 90 Days of Life

For infants from 61 to 90 days of age the criteria have loosened a bit, where this age group previously would also have gotten a full sepsis workup. The reason for this is the advent of the Prevnar vaccine against *Streptococcus.* The vaccine is administered at 2, 4, and 6 months, and it seems to have decreased the incidence of SBI in infants older than 2 months.

A reasonable strategy for this age group is to obtain a basic workup including CBC with differential, blood culture, UA, and urine culture. If the child appears well a lumbar puncture (LP) can be foregone. An LP should be performed if the WBC count is greater than 15 or if a bandemia greater than 10% exists. It is important to remember that infants should not receive antibiotics unless an LP is performed. This is to avoid partially treated meningitis, which could have serious sequelae if it goes on unrecognized. If the child looks well and the labs are normal, he or she can be discharged home without an LP or antibiotics, provided that follow-up can be assured within 24 hours.

LITERATURE REFERENCE

Does RSV-positivity obviate the need for sepsis evaluation in infants less than 60 days of age?

The evaluation of fever in infants < 60 days of age is difficult due to the presence of an immature immune system coupled with localizing signs and symptoms of infection that are often absent. Although SBI occurs in approximately 10% of febrile infants in this age group, many infants present to the ED with fever and the clinical syndrome of bronchiolitis. Levine et al. evaluated 1,248 infants <60 days of age who were febrile (temperature >38°C). Respiratory syncitial virus (RSV)-positive infants had a lower rate of SBI when compared with RSV-negative infants (7.0% vs 12.5%). In the RSV-positive infants, the rate of UTI was still clinically significant at 5.4% (versus 10.1% in the RSV-negative infants). Subgroup analysis by age revealed that the rate of SBI in children <28 days, regardless of RSV status, was not significantly different (10.1% vs 14.2%, p < 0.05). Therefore, a sepsis evaluation is still mandatory in this age group. In the infants between 29 to 60 days of age, there was a statistically significant decline in the rate of SBI in RSV-positive infants (5.5% vs 11.7%, p < 0.05). The authors conclude that the presence of RSV decreases the likelihood of SBI in infants between the age of 29 and 60 days, but that the rate of UTI was still clinically significant, making urine culture an important part of the diagnostic evaluation [**Levine DA et al. *Pediatrics.* 2004;113:1728–1734**].

Should Bronchiolitis Change Your Strategy?

Bronchiolitis is a common viral respiratory illness in infants, especially during winter months. And it is a common source of fever as well. However, good judgment and supporting data show that the presence of clinical bronchiolitis should not alter the workup of fever given the relatively high incidence of SBI coincident with bronchiolitis. Therefore, febrile infants less than 2 months of age still require a full sepsis workup while those between 61 to 90 days receive a basic workup.

KEY POINTS

- The workup of pediatric fever depends on multiple factors
  - Age of the patient
  - "Toxic" appearance
  - Exposures
  - Immune status
  - Presence of source identified on physical examination
- All ill-appearing children should be placed on a monitor, given supplemental oxygen, and have intravenous access obtained
- Blood, urine, and CSF cultures should be obtained prior to the administration of broad-spectrum empiric antibiotics
  - Give antibiotics prior to LP if suspicion for meningitis is high
- Diagnostic evaluation of infants less than 3 months of age with fever should focus on excluding SBI
  - SBI includes meningitis, pneumonia, urinary tract infection, bacteremia, bacterial enteritis, and other skin, bone, and soft-tissue infections
- Neonates (less than 28 days of age) with fever require a full sepsis evaluation, intravenous antibiotics, and admission to the hospital
- Infants between the age of 29 and 60 days should have a complete sepsis evaluation
  - Thereafter may be managed as outpatients after the administration of intramuscular ceftriaxone if they are low risk
  - An alternative strategy is to admit these low-risk infants to the hospital for observation *without* antibiotics
- Well-appearing infants older than 60 days may potentially forgo LP and be treated without antibiotics
  - Basic workup includes CBC with diff, blood culture, UA and culture

FEVER

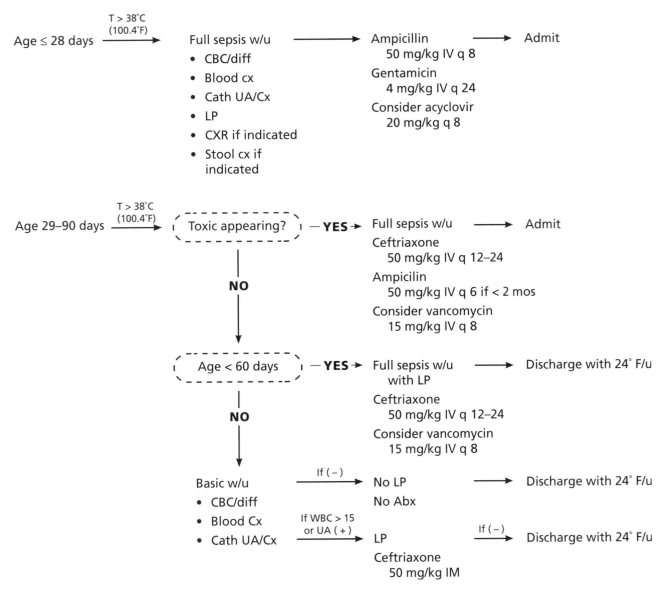

*CXR, chest X-ray; F/u, follow-up; w/u, work-up; Abx, antibiotics; cx, culture

CHAPTER 8

Fever: 3–36 Months

CASE SCENARIO

An 8-month-old female infant presents with her mother to the ED with a chief complaint of fever. The mother reports that the child has been ill for the past 2 days with fever as high as 39.5°C. Today, the patient has seemed fussy and has vomited once. She has had no upper respiratory symptoms and has had no diarrhea. Her vital signs reveal a rectal temperature of 39.5°C, a pulse of 160, a respiratory rate of 28, and a blood pressure of 99/45. Oxygen saturation is normal.

1. From the initial history, what factor is most concerning for serious bacterial infection (SBI)?
   a. Fussiness
   b. Vomiting
   c. Fever of 39.5°C
   d. Absence of diarrhea

Irritability and vomiting are nonspecific findings that are often present with SBI, but can be present in many other illnesses as well. On the other hand, the degree of fever does correlate with the risk of bacterial illness. The mother reports that the child was previously healthy without chronic medical problems or current medications. The family immigrated to the United States from Mexico 2 months ago and the child has received only one set of vaccinations as her pediatrician is trying to "catch her up." Physical examination reveals a consolable infant without abnormalities.

2. Which of the following organisms would be LEAST likely to cause this patient's illness?
   a. *Haemophilus influenzae* type b
   b. *Streptococcus pneumonia*
   c. Group B streptococcus
   d. *Escherichia coli*

The development of childhood vaccines for *Haemophilus influenzae* type b (Hib) and *Streptococcus pneumonia* (pneumococcal heptavalent conjugate vaccine, Prevnar) have caused a dramatic decline in the number of cases of bacteremia in the pediatric population. These vaccines are typically given at 2, 4, and 6 months of age and all three doses are needed for full immunity. *H. influenzae* should still be considered in immigrants to this country. *E. coli* is a common cause of urinary tract infections in infants and can cause bacteremia and sepsis if untreated. Group B strep is a common cause of neonatal sepsis but would be unlikely in an older child. Given the child's lack of immunizations, you decide a diagnostic workup is warranted.

3. Which of the following would be the most appropriate tests to obtain?
   a. Complete blood count (CBC), blood culture, urinalysis (UA), urine culture
   b. CBC, blood culture, UA, urine culture, lumbar puncture (LP)
   c. UA, urine culture
   d. CBC, blood culture

Multiple different strategies exist for the evaluation of a febrile infant of this age. These strategies seek to identify the small subset of patients with occult bacteremia who are at risk to progress to meningitis and/or sepsis. The patient in question should have a CBC, blood culture, UA, and urine culture obtained. LP should be considered in patients with signs of meningitis but is not warranted in this case. In this case, the UA reveals 2+ leukocyte esterase and 50 to 100 white blood cells (WBC)/hpf. The child is discharged on cephalexin and has follow-up arranged for the next day with her pediatrician for a renal ultrasound and vesicoureterogram to rule out congenital anatomic abnormalities.

4. Which of the following would be an appropriate treatment strategy if the child were 4 months old?
   a. CBC, blood culture, UA, urine culture
   b. CBC, blood culture, UA, urine culture, LP
   c. UA, urine culture
   d. CBC, blood culture

The treatment strategy would be the same in this case regardless of the child's age because of his incomplete immunization status. An LP is required in infants greater than 3 months of age only if the child looks ill or if the WBC is greater than 15 or has a significant bandemia. Febrile children older than 6 months can be discharged home without any workup (other than a cath urinalysis for girls < 3 years and uncircumcised boys < 1 year) provided their immunizations are up-to-date, they appear healthy and they have evidence of SBI on examination. It is important however that these children have reliable follow-up within 24 hours.

Answers: 1-c, 2-c, 3-a, 4-a

INITIAL EVALUATION

Fever is not a disease but a sign of underlying illness. Thus, the evaluation should not focus on the fever itself but on its possible etiologies. While parents and caregivers often focus on the fever, it actually is a sign of a healthy immune response to infection. A thorough history and physical examination are essential in determining further evaluation and treatment (see Table 8-1).

Providers are often asked to make an assessment of whether the child is toxic appearing or not. While poorly defined, toxicity generally refers to infants with poor eye contact, poor interactions with parents and the environment, signs of poor perfusion, hypoventilation, hyperventilation, cyanosis or petechiae. While often viral in origin, fever and petechiae can be caused by SBI, including *Neisseria meningitidis*. Any toxic-appearing infant requires immediate evaluation, intravenous access, laboratory evaluation, and treatment with antibiotics.

LITERATURE REFERENCE

 Hot tots with spots—The significance of fever and petechiae

A petechial rash is common in cases of meningococcemia and is caused by the disseminated intravascular coagulation that occurs as a result of overwhelming sepsis. Viral illnesses and streptococcal pharyngitis can also cause petechial rash, which makes evaluation of the highly febrile child with petechiae more difficult. Mandl et al. enrolled 411 patients in a prospective cohort study that was designed to determine the incidence of bacteremia in infants and children with fever and petechiae. They reported a 1.9% incidence of bacteremia or clinical sepsis amongst children aged 0 to 18 years with fever >38°C and petechiae, all of whom were clinically ill appearing. A peripheral WBC of <5,000/mm^3 or >15,000/mm^3 was associated with serious bacterial disease and all children with meningococcemia had true purpura as well as petechiae. They concluded that it was possible to manage most cases as outpatient as long as they had normal laboratory values and were clinically stable during a period of observation in the emergency department [**Mandl KD et al. *J Pediatr.* 1997;131:398–404**].

TABLE 8-1 Physical findings and associated infection	
History & Physical	**Infection**
Cough, runny nose	URI
Cough, tachypnea	Pneumonia
Otalgia, TM fullness, or pus	Otitis media
Sore throat, exudates, lymphadenopathy	Pharyngitis
Lethargy, irritability	Sepsis, meningitis

INFANTS AND TODDLERS (3–36 MONTHS)

Occult bacteremia is defined as evidence of bacteria in the blood with no evidence of toxicity or sepsis and no focal findings on examination. Occult bacteremia was initially described in this age group of infants with fever and mild upper respiratory tract changes. This was found in the 1960s to be secondary to transient *S. pneumoniae* infection and often cleared on its own without therapy, affecting up to 4% to 10% of infants with fever. Studies in the 1970s and 1980s revealed the three most common pathogens of bacteremia to be *S. pneumonia, Haemophilus influenzae* type B and *N. meningitidis*, with small amounts of *Salmonella* and *Staphylococcus aureus*. Patients may present with fever or in the setting of a febrile seizure. Without therapy, bacteremia usually resolves spontaneously but can lead to serious illness including septic arthritis, sepsis, or meningitis. The predilection to seed distant sites differs depending on the organism involved. *H. influenzae* type B bacteremia has up to a 20% risk of disseminated infection, including meningitis. *N. meningitidis* bacteremia has up to 50% risk of disseminated infection, including sepsis and meningitis. In contrast, pneumococcemia has only about a 5% risk of meningitis and focal complications.

In 1993, an important treatment guideline outlined the risk of bacteremia and treatment to prevent its sequelae. It recommended children 3 to 36 months of age with fever > 39°C and whose WBC count >15,000/μL should be treated with antibiotics pending blood culture results. Patients were traditionally given a dose of intramuscular ceftriaxone 50 mg/kg after blood cultures and instructed to see their doctor for follow-up the next day for a repeat dose of ceftriaxone. This guideline has driven the treatment of fever without source for the last decade and helped prevent adverse outcomes from missed cases of bacteremia. Current medical advances make these treatment guidelines outdated.

With the introduction of *H. influenza* type B (Hib) immunization in the early 1990s, the rate of invasive Hib disease decreased markedly to a rate in one study of only 1.6% out of almost 10,000 blood cultures. Pneumococcus then became the major cause of bacteremia, accounting for greater than 90% of cases of bacteremia. The epidemiology of bacteremia in febrile infants continues to evolve after the introduction of the heptavalent conjugate pneumococcal vaccine (Prevnar) in February 2000. Since its introduction, there has been close to an 80% reduction in invasive pneumococcal disease in children under 2 years of age as discussed in the previous chapter. In children 3 to 36 months of age with high fever, leukocytosis, and prior Hib and Prevnar immunization, the rate of bacteremia is less than 1%. With the decline in invasive disease due to Hib and pneumococcus, the evaluation and treatment of infants aged 3 to 36 months has also evolved (see the algorithm at the end of this chapter).

A CBC, blood culture, UA, and urine culture should be obtained in infants 3 to 6 months of age with a fever greater than 39°C. The reason for this basic workup is that the Prevnar vaccine is given at 2, 4, and 6 months; therefore, full immunization is attained after 6 months of age. CBC and blood culture are not necessary in well-appearing infants older than 6 months who have received three doses of Hib and Prevnar. In this age group however, UA is still an important part of the evaluation as well as a urine culture to rule out UTI. This is particularly important in girls under 3 years and in uncircumcised boys under 1 year of age.

FEVER IN IMMUNOCOMPROMISED CHILDREN

Fever in an immunocompromised child is sepsis until proven otherwise. Defects in immune function can be congenital (e.g., patients with primary immune deficiencies), or acquired (e.g., patients undergoing chemotherapy for cancer). Neutropenia in children is defined as an absolute WBC count of less than 1,500/μL. The causative organisms in immunocompromised patients are different from those in normal infants (see Box 8-1). Coagulase-negative staphylococci, *S. aureus*, and alpha-hemolytic streptococci are the most common cultured organisms in neutropenic patients. Important pathogens to consider include *Pseudomonas aeruginosa*, gram-negative rods, Pneumocystis carinii (PCP), and fungal infections. Patients with indwelling catheters are at risk for colonization with bacteria and line sepsis. Infections common to immunocompromised hosts should be sought, including mucositis, sinusitis, cutaneous lesions, or perirectal abscesses.

Patients should have a CBC with manual differential and blood cultures from central venous catheter lumens as well from a peripheral vein. UA and urine culture should be obtained. If neutropenia is suspected, the goal should be antibiotic administration within 1 hour of presentation without waiting for lab results. Antibiotic therapy should be broad. Common regimens include cefepime monotherapy or ceftazidime and an aminoglycoside to cover gram-negative and gram-positive organisms, as well as pseudomonas. Vancomycin is added for increasing gram-positive coverage (especially coagulase-negative staphylococcus) for

---

BOX 8-1   Common pathogens in immunocompromised children

Bacterial
  E. coli
  Pseudomonas aeruginosa
  Enterobacter
  Klebsiella
  S. aureus
  Staphylococcus, coagulase-negative
  S. pneumonia
  Streptococcus viridians
  Enterococcus faecalis
  Bacillus
  H. influenzae

Virus
  Varicella-zoster
  Herpes simplex virus (HSV)
  Epstein-Barr virus (EBV)
  Cytomegalovirus (CMV)
  Enteroviruses
  Respiratory viruses

Fungal
  Candida albicans
  Aspergillus
  Cryptococcus
  Pneumocystis carinii

Protozoa
  Toxoplasmosis

---

patients with indwelling catheters. Neutropenic and otherwise immunocompromised children require admission for continued broad-spectrum treatment until cultures grow a specific organism.

FEVER IN SICKLE CELL ANEMIA

Sickle cell patients can in effect be considered immunocompromised given their increased risk for developing SBI. The leading cause of death among children with sickle cell disease is pneumococcal sepsis. Sickle cell patients have functional asplenia due to autoinfarction, resulting in the inability to clear encapsulated bacteria from the blood. Sickle cell patients are at risk for pneumonia and bacteremia caused by *S. pneumonia* and Hib, bacteremia and osteomyelitis caused by *Salmonella*, and pyelonephritis caused by *E. coli*. Sickle cell patients are also at high risk for aplastic crises after parvovirus infection. Acute chest syndrome, with features of fever, chest pain, cough, abdominal pain, and hypoxia affects about 40% of sickle cell patients and occurs most commonly in children.

History should focus on the presence of fever, pain, cough, difficulty breathing, headache, and hydration status. A history of acute chest pain crises, splenic sequestration, and stroke or transfusion dependence are indicative of more severe sickle cell disease. Compliance with daily antibiotic prophylaxis, usually penicillin, should be assessed as well as current immunization status for Prevnar, pneumococcal vaccine polyvalent (Pneumovax) if greater than 2 years of age, meningococcus, and influenza. Patients under 5 years of age who take daily penicillin have an over 80% reduction in pneumococcal sepsis.

A CBC with manual differential, reticulocyte count and blood culture should be obtained in these patients. Antibiotics should not be delayed awaiting CBC results and should consist of ceftriaxone 50 mg/kg given within 1 hour of presentation. A chest x-ray is indicated to evaluate for acute chest syndrome if the child has chest pain. Admission should be considered for continued antibiotic treatment and for observation for possible complications of vaso-occlusive crises, including acute chest syndrome.

KEY POINTS

- Fever is a sign of underlying illness
  - Thorough history and physical examination are necessary for investigation
- Evaluation is dictated by toxic appearance
  - Poor eye contact, poor interactions with parents and the environment, poor perfusion, hypo- or hyperventilation, cyanosis or petechiae
  - Requires full sepsis workup including CBC and blood cultures, UA and urine cultures, cerebrospinal fluid (CSF) with gram stain and cultures
  - Broad-spectrum antibiotics such as ceftriaxone, vancomycin, and clindamycin
- In non-toxic appearing children, workup is tailored
  - Febrile (T > 39°C) infants 3 to 6 months require a "basic" workup
  - CBC and blood cultures, UA and urine cultures
  - After 6-months workup can be focused based on presentation
  - UA and urine culture should be obtained for girls < 3 years and uncircumcised boys < 1 year if no other obvious infection is identified
- Immunocompromised children and those with sickle cell disease require antibiotics within 1 hour of presentation

FEVER

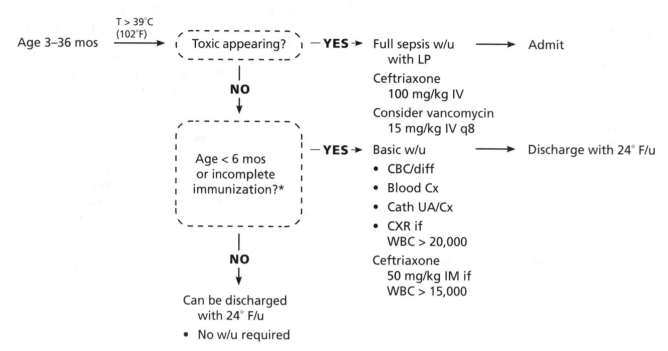

*Complete immunization includes Prevnar and Hib at 2, 4, 6 months

CHAPTER 9

Altered Mental Status

CASE SCENARIO

You are working in the emergency department when a young mother brings her 16-month-old daughter in for evaluation. She reports that the child had been crying and irritable for most of the day but that she had finally succeeded in getting her to go down for her nap at about 3 p.m. At 5 p.m., she went in to wake her and had a hard time so she called her pediatrician and was referred in for evaluation.

1. You enter the room to find a toddler who is somnolent and moans when you examine her. What do you do?
   a. Check a fingerstick blood glucose
   b. Establish IV access, supply oxygen via a non rebreather mask, and place on a monitor
   c. Empirically administer naloxone IV
   d. STAT head CT

All of the above answers are appropriate for this case but your first priority should be to establish IV access, administer oxygen, and get the patient on a monitor. Hypoglycemia is an important cause of altered mental status (AMS), especially in known diabetics or in toddlers who can have ketotic hypoglycemia with prolonged fasts. Naloxone is indicated because prescription drug overdose is relatively common in the toddler age group due to their propensity to put anything and everything into their mouths. You document normal blood glucose and note no response to naloxone. The patient's vital signs on the monitor include a heart rate of 70, a blood pressure of 125/80, a respiratory rate of 20, a temperature of 36.5°C, and an oxygen saturation of 100% on oxygen.

2. What is your next step?
   a. Send blood for chemistries, serum toxicologic screening, complete blood count (CBC), blood culture
   b. Obtain a computed tomography (CT) of the head
   c. Perform a lumbar puncture
   d. Perform a physical examination

Although the workup for AMS often involves imaging studies and laboratory evaluation, the first step is to perform a thorough physical examination. The answer is often found in the history, vital signs, and physical examination. She has no evidence of head trauma, her neck is supple without meningismus, her heart and lung examinations are normal, her abdominal examination reveals no tenderness, and she is warm and well perfused. Besides the relative hypertension and bradycardia, you note some bruising on the child's shins and arms, and a small circular lesion on the forearm that looks like a burn. During your examination, the child's breathing pattern becomes a bit more erratic with periodic pauses and snoring. You attempt to arouse her with nailbed pressure without success.

3. What is the most appropriate action?
   a. Obtain a head CT
   b. Immediate endotracheal intubation
   c. Call neurosurgery to consult
   d. Call social work to consult

All of these interventions are indicated but your first priority should be to adhere to the airway, breathing, circulation (ABCs) and intubate the patient. Your physical examination has narrowed your differential considerably and the presence of diffuse bruising and what looks like a cigarette burn, make nonaccidental head trauma (i.e., child abuse) a significant concern. You call neurosurgery and social work and then whisk the child off to CT scan where you find a frontal hemorrhagic intracranial contusion and evidence of cerebral edema. The child is admitted to the intensive care unit (ICU) and further workup reveals the presence of posterior rib fractures, retinal hemorrhages, and multiple long bone fractures of various ages, all indicative of abuse.

Answers: 1-b, 2-d, 3-b

DEFINITION

AMS can be broadly categorized into two distinct presentations: patients presenting with a decreased level of consciousness or patients presenting with an acute confusional state (delirium). As such, it represents a sign of disease rather than a disease entity in and of itself. Although there are literally hundreds of possible causes of alteration in mental status, they all share the common final pathway of either bilateral cerebral hemispheric dysfunction or brainstem (reticular activating system) dysfunction. Diseases or conditions affecting either of these two areas have the potential to cause alterations in consciousness, and because the list of possible etiologies is long, a systematic approach to each patient is a necessity.

ETIOLOGY

There are almost as many ways to approach a patient with AMS as there are causes for AMS. A systems-based approach is presented in Box 9-1, where the differential diagnosis is broken up by body system. For example, neurologic causes of mental status change include seizure, stroke, and shunt malfunction, while cardiac etiologies include ischemia, congestive heart failure, and arrhythmia. Infectious etiologies include meningitis, encephalitis, sepsis, and bacteremia. Pulmonary causes include things such as hypoxia or hypercarbia. Inborn errors of metabolism causing hyperammonemia or metabolic acidosis, and endocrinopathies (such as diabetes and Graves' disease) frequently can cause change in level of consciousness. There are many toxic ingestions that can present with AMS including drugs of abuse (cocaine, hallucinogens, opiates), anticholinergics, sedative hypnotics, and the alcohols. Several environmental exposures are potential etiologies including heat stroke, hypothermia or carbon monoxide poisoning.

BOX 9-1　Etiologies of altered mental status by system

Neurologic
Seizure or postictal state
Stroke
Ventriculoperitoneal shunt obstruction
Intracranial hemorrhage (subdural, subarachnoid, epidural)
Trauma, including abuse
Mass (neoplasm, abscess)
Psychiatric disease

Cardiac
Myocardial ischemia
Congestive heart failure
Cardiac arrhythmia (bradycardia or tachycardia associated with poor perfusion)

Infectious
Meningitis
Encephalitis
Sepsis
Pneumonia
Toxic shock syndrome
Bacteremia/meningococcemia
Hemolytic uremic syndrome

Pulmonary
Hypoxia
Hypercarbia
Respiratory failure
Pulmonary embolus

Gastrointestinal
Hepatic failure
GI bleeding
Intussusception
Volvulus
Necrotizing enterocolitis
Malrotation
Pyloric stenosis
Nutritional deficiencies

Endocrine/Metabolic
Hyper/Hypoglycemia
Thyroid
Adrenal
Electrolyte disturbances (particularly hyponatremia)
Inborn errors of metabolism (hyperammonemia, metabolic acidosis)

Hematologic
Anemia

Renal
Uremia

Toxic
Opiates
Benzodiazepines
Barbiturates
Anticholinergics
Anticonvulsants
Antidepressants
Cardiac medications (beta-blockers, calcium-channel blockers, digoxin)
Psychotropic drugs
Aspirin
Tylenol
Alcohols (ethanol, methanol, ethylene glycol, isopropyl alcohol)
Lead encephalopathy
Heavy metal poisoning

Environmental exposure
Heatstroke and hyperthermia
Hypothermia
Altitude sickness (high-altitude cerebral edema)
Carbon monoxide poisoning

As the above discussion illustrates, there are myriad potential etiologies for AMS and the goal should be to have a systematic "mental algorithm" to run through so as not to miss the specific cause for your patient.

TREATMENT

General Approach

The patient with AMS can be a complex and challenging scenario due to the multiple possible etiologies. Your initial approach to the patient should be to support the ABCs while using historical, vital sign, and physical examination clues to root out the cause for the change in level of consciousness. While the history you are able to obtain from the patient with change in mental status will be limited, valuable clues to the diagnosis may come from parents, friends or

Emergency Medical Service (EMS) providers who were at the scene. Often, EMS providers will bring pill bottles or chemicals found at the scene if a toxic ingestion is suspected.

Resuscitation: ABCs, IV-Oxygen-Monitor

The initial approach to the patient with AMS should focus on support of the ABCs. It is absolutely critical that the brain have oxygen, blood flow, and a source of glucose at all times. If the patient has a Glasgow coma scale (GCS) of 8 or less (see Table 9-1), is failing to oxygenate or ventilate, or has lost protective airway reflexes, then intubation is indicated. Although the GCS was initially designed and validated in trauma patients, it can be used as a general indicator of level of consciousness in medical patients as well. Quality of perfusion should be assessed after evaluation of the airway and breathing. Hypotension should be treated with intravenous fluids or vasopressors to ensure adequate perfusion. These maneuvers may serve to treat the change in mental status if it is due to hypoxia, hypercarbia, or hypoperfusion while allowing time for further diagnostic evaluation. All patients should have IV access, be given supplemental oxygen if they don't meet criteria for endotracheal intubation, and be placed on a cardiac monitor.

TABLE 9-1 Glasgow coma scale	
Eye opening	
Spontaneous	4
To speech	3
To pain	2
None	1
Verbal response	
Oriented	5
Confused conversation	4
Inappropriate words	3
Incomprehensible sounds	2
None	1
Best motor response	
Obeys commands	6
Localizes pain	5
Withdrawal to pain	4
Decorticate posturing	3
Decerebrate posturing	2
None	1

Empiric Treatment with the "Coma Cocktail"

Once the ABCs have been addressed, attention should be placed on identifying and treating readily reversible causes of AMS. Glucose and naloxone are together considered the coma cocktail and empiric treatment with these agents should be considered in cases of undifferentiated mental status changes (see Table 9-2). Glucose is given as D25 (25% glucose solution) at a dose of 0.5 to 1 gram/kg IV. Hypoglycemia can cause general mental status depression or coma, focal neurologic findings that mimic stroke, or even seizures. Prompt restoration of circulating glucose is critical to prevent permanent neurologic sequelae. Bradypnea, hypoxia, and hypotension are the classic characteristics of the opiate toxidrome, which can be successfully reversed with naloxone. Naloxone is given in a dose of 0.1 mg/kg IV and may actually obviate the need for intubation in cases of opiate overdose.

Vital Signs are Vital

Once the ABCs have been stabilized and the coma cocktail given, attention is given to decoding the vital signs. The vitals are the most critical portion of the physical examination and often give clues to the etiology of AMS (see Table 9-3). Heart rate, blood pressure, respiratory rate, oxygen saturation, and rectal temperature should be obtained at the beginning of every patient encounter and reassessed frequently during the resuscitation. Tachycardia may herald hypovolemia, sepsis, or drug ingestion as a cause of mental status changes. Bradycardia is common with severe hypoxia or beta-blocker overdose. Hypotension may be due to hypovolemia or sepsis while hypertension is common with sympathomimetic drug overdose (e.g., cocaine). Tachypnea may indicate metabolic acidosis due to diabetic ketoacidosis or methanol ingestion. Hypoxia may be due to pneumonia or cyanide poisoning. Certain patterns of vital sign abnormalities can suggest specific etiologies such as the bradycardia and hypertension that accompany increased intracranial pressure or the tachycardia, fever, and hypotension that herald the onset of sepsis.

TABLE 9-2	Elements of the coma cocktail
Drug	**Dose**
Glucose	0.5 to 1 g/kg IV/IO (2 to 4 mL/kg of D25, 5 to 10 mL/kg of D10, 10 to 20 mL/kg of D5)
Naloxone	0.1 mg/kg IV

TABLE 9-3	Vital signs as a clue to altered mental status
Fever/Hyperthermia	Infection, heatstroke, neuroleptic malignant syndrome, thyroid storm
Hypothermia	Exposure, sepsis, myxedema, coma
Tachycardia	Sepsis, hypovolemia, sympathomimetic toxidrome, anticholinergic toxidrome
Bradycardia	Increased intracranial pressure, beta-blocker overdose, calcium-channel blocker overdose, hypoxia
Hypertension	Sympathomimetic toxidrome, intracranial hemorrhage
Hypotension	Sepsis, hypovolemia, opiate toxidrome, sedative hypnotic toxidrome
Tachypnea	Acidosis (diabetic ketoacidosis, lactic acidosis), aspirin overdose, hypoxia
Hypoxia	Pneumonia, pulmonary embolus, congestive heart failure

Physical Examination

Once the vital signs have been decoded, a thorough and complete physical examination should be completed. Often, clues to the etiology of AMS can be found on examination (see Table 9-4). In children, the examination should focus on signs of trauma, infection, and drug ingestion as these are the three most common broad categories of illnesses causing AMS. Trauma may be heralded by scalp hematomas, palpable skull fractures, or CSF otorhinorrhea. Retinal hemorrhages may indicate child abuse (see Box 9-2). Meningismus, petechiae, or purpura can occur with meningitis and meningococcemia, while rales may indicate pneumonia. Drug ingestions can cause pinpoint pupils (opiates), mydriasis (cocaine), or dry mucous membranes (diphenhydramine) while irritant dermatitis around the lips and nose may be an indicator of huffing (inhalation of volatile hydrocarbons). It is also critically important to completely expose the patient and thoroughly examine the diaper area and genitals in infants for signs of trauma or infection.

Treatment and Workup Go Hand in Hand

The workup for AMS will in most cases involve laboratory tests and diagnostic imaging. It is important

TABLE 9-4 Physical examination clues to altered mental status

Mydriasis	Anticholinergic (e.g., diphenhydramine) or sympathomimetic (e.g., cocaine) toxidrome
Miosis	Opiate overdose
Unequal pupils	Intracranial hemorrhage or mass
Scleral icterus	Hepatic encephalopathy
Dry mucous membranes	Dehydration, sepsis, anticholinergic toxidrome
Nuchal rigidity	Meningitis, subarachnoid hemorrhage
Rash	Meningococcemia, toxic shock syndrome
Bruising	Child abuse, trauma
Heart murmur	Endocarditis, anemia
Melena or guaiac positive stool	Intussusception

BOX 9-3 Laboratory and diagnostic imaging used in the workup of altered mental status

- Blood glucose
- Basic chemistries (sodium, potassium, chloride, bicarbonate, anion gap, blood urea nitrogen (BUN), creatinine, magnesium, calcium, phosphorus)
- CBC
- UA
- Blood and urine cultures
- Lumbar puncture
- Serum ammonia
- Blood and urine toxicology screens
- ECG
- Chest radiograph
- Head CT scan

to cast a broad net and be relatively liberal in regard to diagnostic testing when working up AMS (see Box 9-3), although it is often necessary to begin therapy before a diagnosis is made or results of blood work are available. Broad-coverage empiric antibiotics should be given to any critically ill child in whom infection, particularly meningitis, is a concern. Ceftriaxone 100 mg/kg IV for infants and children older than 28 days or ampicillin and gentamicin for neonates are acceptable empiric regimens. A head CT is indicated if there is suspicion for traumatic etiology, focal findings on neurologic exam, or no clear toxic or metabolic cause for the alteration in consciousness.

Serum and urine toxicology screens may be useful diagnostically though many drugs of abuse (e.g.,

methylenedioxymethamphetamine [MDMA], gamma-hydroxybutyrate [GHB]) do not show up on routine panels. Blood chemistries may be useful to evaluate for hyponatremia, metabolic acidosis, or renal failure. A complete blood count and blood culture may be useful if systemic infection is suspected. Liver function tests and serum ammonia levels are indicated if hepatic failure or inborn error of metabolism is high on the differential. An ECG can be useful in diagnosing arrhythmia or myocarditis while chest radiographs can show pneumonia or cardiomegaly, which may offer a diagnostic clue.

DISPOSITION

Most patients presenting with AMS will be admitted to the hospital for further workup and treatment. Simple hypoglycemia that responds to glucose therapy or patients with AMS due to seizure without concern for CNS trauma or infection can potentially be managed as outpatients.

KEY POINTS

- Potential etiologies of AMS are numerous
- History, vital signs, and physical examination are often the keys to diagnosis
- Obtain careful history from friends, family, or EMS providers
- Completely undress each patient so as not to miss rashes or trauma

BOX 9-2 Injury patterns concerning for child abuse

- Traction alopecia (parent pulling hair of child)
- Metaphyseal chip fractures
- Multiple injuries at various stages of healing
- Posterior rib fractures
- Intracranial hemorrhage without external signs of trauma (shaken baby syndrome)
- Retinal hemorrhages
- Loop shaped bruises (electrical cord)
- Immersion burns
- Cigarette burns

- Approach each patient systematically
  - ABCs, history and physical examination (H&P), vital signs, laboratory and radiographic studies
- "Coma cocktail" if suspected hypoglycemia or opiate overdose
- Have a systems-based approach to the differential diagnosis
  - CNS, infectious, toxicologic
- Be liberal with laboratory testing and diagnostic imaging, especially head CT
- Treat for meningitis early in patients without another obvious source
- Admit for further workup

CHAPTER 10

Head Trauma

CASE SCENARIO

You are working in the ED when paramedics bring in a 2-year-old child who fell 6 feet off a bunk bed at home. His parents heard a "thud" and ran into the room to find him unconscious and actively seizing on the hardwood floor. His seizure lasted approximately 60 seconds and he has since been gradually more arousable. Vital signs in the field reveal a blood pressure of 100/60, pulse of 110, respiratory rate of 28, and an oxygen saturation of 100% on a nonrebreather mask. Upon arrival, he is somnolent but arousable.

1. What is your next step?
   a. Check a fingerstick blood glucose
   b. Establish intravenous (IV) access, administer oxygen, and place the patient on a monitor
   c. Administer rectal Valium
   d. Obtain a computed tomography (CT) scan of the head

Your first priority should be to establish IV access, continue oxygen administration, and place him on a monitor. Hypoglycemia is a common cause of seizure but there is nothing from the history to suggest this as the etiology of his presentation. Benzodiazepines are the initial anticonvulsant of choice for acute seizure but this child is not actively seizing. CT of the head is advisable but not until IV-O_2-monitor is established. Although initially more lucid, the child begins to become more somnolent with sonorous respirations and his heart rate drops below 80.

2. What do you do now?
   a. Immediate intubation via rapid sequence techniques
   b. Obtain a stat neurosurgical consult
   c. Take the child immediately to CT scan
   d. Push IV mannitol

All of these actions are appropriate but of first and foremost importance are the airway, breathing, and circulation (ABCs). This child is showing signs of herniation and is losing his ability to maintain a patent airway and breathe. He should be immediately intubated to protect his airway and prevent hypoxia, which is a significant cause of secondary brain injury. The child is successfully intubated and is taken directly to CT.

3. Which of the following is most likely, given the scenario presented?
   a. Diffuse axonal injury
   b. Small subdural hematoma
   c. Traumatic subarachnoid hemorrhage
   d. Epidural hematoma

Although all of these injuries can occur after head trauma, the presence of a lucid interval followed by abrupt clinical deterioration is classic for epidural hematoma. Epidural hematomas occur most commonly with parietal skull fracture and laceration of the middle meningeal artery. Initially, patients may be asymptomatic but as blood accumulates under arterial pressure and displaces brain parenchyma, symptoms develop. If not expeditiously evacuated, herniation, coma, and death rapidly follow. This child had a large epidural noted on the right and was taken to the operating room (OR) where it was evacuated successfully. After 4 days in the intensive care unit (ICU), he made a full recovery.

Answers: 1-b, 2-a, 3-d

EPIDEMIOLOGY

Head injury is the most common cause of death amongst injured children and results in greater than 600,000 ED visits and over $1 billion in medical expenditures each year. The etiology of head trauma death changes as a child ages with nonaccidental trauma being much more common in infants less than 1 year of age. Older children are more likely to sustain a head injury in a motor vehicle collision, a fall, or when struck by a car.

DEFINITION

Primary brain injury involves direct trauma to the brain parenchyma. Prevention of primary brain injury involves public health initiatives such as seat belt and helmet use. Secondary brain injury involves the complex cascade of events that occur after trauma with hypoxia, hypotension, metabolic derangements, release of free radicals, and edema being the major players.

BOX 10-1	Clinical predictors of intracranial injury (ICI)
• Presence of a skull fracture
• Altered mental status
• Head injury without history of trauma
• Younger age
• Inflicted injury
• Focal neurologic findings
• Scalp swelling

Head trauma runs the gamut from devastating neurologic injury and major mechanism trauma to the minor bumps and bruises of childhood (see Table 10-1). The vast majority of pediatric patients with head trauma do not sustain an intracranial injury (ICI), but there are certain high-risk criteria that are predictive of significant injury (see Box 10-1). The Glasgow coma scale (GCS) can be useful in rapidly assessing the severity of head injury (see Table 9.1). Severe head trauma is defined as a GCS of 3 to 8, while moderate head trauma is a GCS of 9 to 13. Minor head trauma is defined as a history of head trauma, with or without clinical signs of blunt trauma to the scalp, in a patient who is alert or awakens to light touch or voice (i.e., GCS score of 14 to 15). Despite a normal neurologic examination, the incidence of ICI in children less than 2 years of age with minor head trauma is 3% to 6%.

TABLE 10-1	Head injury patterns
Type	**Significance**
Linear skull fracture	Marker of intracranial injury (ICI) presence mandates head CT
Depressed skull fracture	Any significant degree of depression may need surgical elevation
Growing fracture	Meningeal tissue herniates into fracture causing erosion of edges over time
Epidural hematoma	May have a lucid interval prior to clinical deterioration
Subdural hematoma	Should raise suspicion of shaken baby syndrome in young children
Subarachnoid hemorrhage	Typically associated with other ICIs
Cerebral contusion	"Bruising" of cortex, often with significant neurologic deficits at the time of presentation
Diffuse axonal injury	Shear injury from acceleration/deceleration injury, poor prognosis

TREATMENT

General Approach

After head injury, initial management should focus on preventing secondary brain injury. Patients with severe head injury or those who are at high risk (see Box 10-1) should be managed in a manner similar to any other critically ill patient with ABCs and IV-O_2-monitor. Patients with hypoxia and hypotension after head trauma have a two-fold mortality, emphasizing the critical importance of airway management and circulatory support.

Indications for immediate intubation after head injury include apnea, hypoxia and absence of protective airway reflexes. Endotracheal intubation should also be strongly considered in patients with a GCS of 8 or less. Patients with moderate head injury also are at high risk for significant ICI, but are not routinely intubated unless they clinically deteriorate. After ABCs and IV-O_2-monitor, these patients should have a directed history and physical examination, and diagnostic imaging should be arranged. In the setting of minor head injury, a detailed history and thorough physical examination should be done looking for any of the high-risk criteria mentioned previously.

Diagnostic Imaging

Non-contrasted CT scanning is the diagnostic modality of choice in moderate to severe head trauma patients. This technology is readily available, fast, and accurate in diagnosing acute injury. Although magnetic resonance imaging (MRI) offers more detailed imaging of the brain parenchyma, it takes much longer to perform, is not as readily available, is less sensitive for acute bleeding, and typically involves transport of the patient away from the ED for prolonged periods.

There is little controversy in the diagnostic algorithm for moderate to severe head trauma (i.e., address ABCs and rapid CT scan), but the same is far from true for cases of mild head trauma. The vast majority of children presenting to the ED for head trauma have a normal neurologic examination and are classified as minor. Obtaining a CT scan on all patients would expose children unnecessarily to ionizing radiation, not to mention that many patients require procedural sedation prior to scanning which has its own inherent risks.

Children greater than 2 years of age with minor head trauma, a normal neurologic examination, and loss of consciousness (LOC) less than 1 minute in duration can safely be observed without imaging. If a longer duration of unconsciousness is present, the child is amnestic, has repeated vomiting, or an abnormal neurologic examination, imaging should be obtained. The younger the patient, the more difficult it is to clinically assess the severity of injury and the lower the threshold should be for imaging (see Table 10-2). Children less than 2 years of age are at higher risk for ICI after minor head trauma, making imaging more important.

Plain x-rays of the skull still have utility in the workup of head injury, even in this day of rapid and easily-accessible CT scanning. The utility of skull films is highest in the neurologically normal child who is greater than 12 months of age who has sustained

TABLE 10-2 Imaging recommendations for children less than 2 years of age

Risk group	Imaging recommendation
High risk Altered mental status Focal neurologic findings Depressed or basilar skull fracture Seizure Irritability Acute skull fracture Bulging fontanel Vomiting ≥5 times or >6 h LOC >1 min	CT scan
Intermediate risk with signs of brain injury Vomiting 3 to 4 times LOC <1 min History of lethargy or irritability Caretaker concern Nonacute skull fracture	CT scan or skull radiograph with clinical observation for 4 to 6 hours after trauma
Higher force mechanism (e.g., MVC or falls >3 to 4 feet) Large, boggy, nonfrontal scalp hematoma Fall onto hard surface Unwitnessed trauma Vague or no history of trauma	CT scan mandated if skull radiograph positive for fracture
Low risk Low energy mechanism No signs or symptoms More than 2 hours from injury Older age more reassuring (age >12 months)	Discharge home without imaging or need for observation

LOC, loss of consciousness; MVC, motor vehicle crash

head trauma with external evidence of trauma (e.g., big skull hematoma) but no signs of ICI on examination. A good example would be a 16-month-old toddler with head trauma and a parietal hematoma, but who is running around the ED. In the absence of signs of increased ICP with negative skull films, a period of observation is reasonable to avoid having to sedate a child for a CT scan.

Brain Specific Therapy

Beyond general resuscitative efforts and attention to the ABCs, options exist for patients with severe head injury and signs of increased intracranial pressure (ICP). Increases in ICP can be provoked by hypercarbia,

Physical signs that should concern you

Proving yet again that there is utility to the physical exam, Greenes et al. found that certain clinical features predicted an increased risk of skull fracture and ICI in asymptomatic children after head injury. They prospectively enrolled 422 children less than 2 years of age after head trauma and found that larger hematomas, those located in the parietal or temporal region, and younger children were more likely to have skull fractures and ICI [Greenes DS, Schutzman SA. *Pediatr Emerg Care.* 2001;17(2):88–92].

hypoxia, hyperthermia, inadequate sedation, or noxious stimuli such as suctioning, and these parameters should be corrected before proceeding further. Cerebral perfusion pressure (mean arterial pressure minus ICP) should be maintained at greater than 40 mm Hg in infants and greater than 70 mm Hg in older children.

ICP Monitoring

Children with severe brain injury should have an ICP monitor placed. Ideally, a ventriculostomy catheter is used that allows for simultaneous ICP monitoring and removal of CSF if needed.

Osmotherapy

Diuretic therapy with mannitol (0.5 to 1 gm/kg IV) can be used as a rescue measure to decrease cerebral blood volume. Care should be taken in patients with extracranial injuries as hypotension may accompany mannitol therapy. Alternatively, 3% saline (hypertonic saline) may be given in boluses of 1 to 2 mL/kg IV in these cases as hypotension is less likely to occur.

Hyperventilation

Hyperventilation to a carbon dioxide partial pressure (Pco_2) of 30 to 35 mm Hg results in a transient decrease in cerebral blood volume and ICP. More aggressive hyperventilation can be used as a last ditch effort pending surgical decompression but is not routinely recommended due to the risk of rebound increases in ICP.

Barbiturates

Barbiturates decrease cerebral metabolism and are indicated in cases of severe head trauma with increased ICP. Pentobarbital is given as a bolus followed by a continuous infusion with the dose titrated to burst suppression on electroencephalogram (EEG). Patients who receive barbiturates by definition require intubation.

Seizure Control

Seizures increase brain metabolism and cerebral blood flow and should be aggressively treated if they occur. Benzodiazepines such as midazolam and lorazepam should be given as first-line agents. Prophylactic antiseizure agents such as phenytoin or fosphenytoin should be administered if there are cortical lesions (e.g., cerebral contusion, subarachnoid hemorrhage).

KEY POINTS

- Primary injury is due to initial impact
- Secondary injury is due to hypoxia, hypoperfusion, free radicals, and edema
  - Aggressively treat hypoxia and hypotension
- Suspect other injuries when evaluating head trauma
  - Complete physical examination required
- CT scanning is the imaging modality of choice in acute head trauma
  - Indicated for all severe and moderate head injury patients
  - Minor head injury may be managed without imaging if low risk
  - The younger the child, the lower the threshold should be to image
- Signs of herniation (hypertension, bradycardia) should be aggressively treated
  - Hyperventilation
  - Osmotic therapy
  - Pentobarbital coma
  - Definitive neurosurgical intervention

CHAPTER 11

Seizure

CASE SCENARIO

A 2-year-old boy arrives by ambulance at the ED after having a suspected seizure at home. Paramedics report that they found the infant at home lying slightly limp in his mother's arms with no visible seizure activity. He was afebrile with normal vital signs for age. He required no intervention en route to the hospital and they note that he has become more vigorous over the 20-minute transport. Upon arrival to the ED, he remains afebrile with a heart rate of 145, blood pressure of 90/55, respiratory rate of 30, and arterial oxygen concentration (SaO_2) of 100% on room air. Physical examination reveals no external evidence of trauma. He is alert and interactive. His pupils are equal and reactive. His neck is supple and his neurologic examination appears normal for age with normal tone and reflexes without clonus. His skin is clear without any evidence for rash or neuro-cutaneous syndromes. The remainder of his examination is nonfocal.

On further questioning, the mother states that he was perfectly well until the morning of presentation when he was eating breakfast and suddenly started to slur his words. Within seconds, he slumped in his chair and began having simultaneous rhythmic jerking motions of all four extremities, causing him to fall to the floor. During this episode, which she estimates lasted 5 minutes, he was not conscious. She does not recall if his eyes were open or deviated during the event. While she was waiting for the ambulance to arrive, the movements stopped and he became still, but he remained unarousable.

1. Based on the above history and physical examination, which tests are indicated in the ED?
   a. Lumbar puncture (LP)
   b. Serum chemistries
   c. Electroencephalogram (EEG)
   d. Computed tomography (CT)
   e. None of the above

A first-time seizure in a child who does not have a fever should raise suspicion for an underlying etiology. In children older than 6 months routine laboratories, head CT, and LP are not necessary for first-time simple seizures; however, close follow-up and outpatient EEG are recommended. Head CT should be performed in children with a suspicion of head trauma, focal seizure activity, focal postictal states that do not rapidly resolve (Todd's paralysis), duration of seizure activity greater than 15 minutes, and persistently altered mental status. Electrolyte disturbances as well as hypoglycemia should also be considered. Hyponatremia is the electrolyte disturbance most often associated with seizures. It can be caused acutely by severe dehydration; it can develop chronically in children with underlying CNS, pulmonary, or renal disease. Hypocalcemia is also associated with seizures. Hypoglycemia is a common cause for seizure, most often insulin-related in children with insulin-dependent diabetes mellitus. Toxic ingestions should always be considered in children with seizure.

Ten minutes later the nurse calls you to the child's room. By the time you make it into the room, you observe a generalized seizure with four extremity tonic-clonic activity. The patient's eyes are opened without a deviated gaze.

2. What is your first step in his management?
   a. Place an IV for lorazepam (Ativan) administration
   b. Give diazepam (Diastat) rectal versed
   c. Apply supplemental 100% oxygen
   d. Obtain a bedside glucose level

During a seizure, there are multiple factors that contribute to hypoxia. There is impaired mechanical ventilation due to the seizure activity and there are increased airway secretions coupled with decreased effective clearance mechanisms. There is also a significantly increased demand for oxygen by the body due to the increased metabolic activity of the muscles and brain. Therefore, as with any emergent situation, the airway should be your first priority and 100% oxygen via a nonrebreather mask should be applied. It is also important to ensure the patient's safety by placing pillows around his head and making sure he does not fall off the bed.

The seizure persists for over 2 minutes. He is maintaining his oxygen saturation with supplemental oxygen via a face mask. You anticipate that he will need pharmacotherapy to break his seizure.

3. Which therapy is preferable at this point?
    a. Administration of Ativan 0.1 mg/kg once IV is established
    b. Administer rectal Valium (Diastat) 0.5 mg/kg
    c. Administer phenytoin 20 mg/kg IV
    d. Administer phenobarbital 20 mg/kg IV

Rectal diazepam gel (Diastat) is a good medication to use at home or in the field as it is easy to administer and does not require IV access. Lorazepam administered IV is preferable in the ED because it has a more rapid onset of action. Diazepam can also be administered IV. Both medications are highly effective at terminating seizure activity. Long-acting antiepileptic drugs (AEDs) such as phenytoin (Dilantin) and phenobarbital are not indicated at this early phase of this patient's care.

4. You obtain IV access and administer lorazepam (Ativan) 0.1 mg/kg. After 1 minute, he continues to seize. What is your next step?
    a. Repeat lorazepam 0.1 mg/kg IV
    b. Administer rectal Valium (Diastat) 0.5 mg/kg
    c. Administer phenytoin 20 mg/kg IV
    d. Administer phenobarbital 20 mg/kg IV
    e. None of the above

While both lorazepam and diazepam have a rapid onset of action, they both on average take approximately 2 to 3 minutes to end seizure activity. Therefore, no further drugs should be administered until approximately 5 minutes following the initial dose. While waiting for the benzodiazepine to take effect, you obtain a glucose which is normal. You also send a complete blood count (CBC) and electrolytes including a blood urea nitrogen (BUN) and creatinine. The monitor indicates that he remains tachycardic with a heart rate of 160 and his blood pressure is elevated at 130/90. His temperature has risen to 103°F.

5. Which of the following laboratory findings is not consistent with status epilepticus?
    a. Metabolic acidosis
    b. Respiratory acidosis
    c. Hyperkalemia
    d. Hypokalemia
    e. Leukocytosis

Seizure activity which extends beyond 30 minutes, or three consecutive seizures without interim regaining of consciousness, is referred to as status epilepticus and is associated with several serious systemic findings. However, even prior to the 30-minute mark, multiple abnormalities can be seen in the blood as a result of generalized tonic-clonic seizure activity. Metabolic acidosis results from vigorous muscle contraction, anaerobic metabolism, and lactate production. Respiratory acidosis results from hypoventilation due to uncoordinated diaphragmatic contractions. Hyperkalemia, not hypokalemia, can also be found with levels proportional to the degree of acidosis, which results in cellular excretion of potassium in exchange for hydrogen ions. Leukocytosis is a result of white blood cell demargination in response to the severe physiologic stress associated with seizure activity. Similarly, the catecholamine surge results in tachycardia and hypertension. The hyperpyrexia results from the seizure activity as well and is difficult to differentiate from fever of infectious etiology. Naturally, meningitis is a concern with fever and seizure.

Approximately 5 minutes following his first dose of Ativan, he is still seizing. His oxygen saturation remains greater than 95% on oxygen. He continues to be tachycardic and hypertensive.

6. What is your next step?
   a. Repeat lorazepam 0.1 mg/kg IV
   b. Administer rectal Valium (Diastat) 0.5 mg/kg
   c. Administer fosphenytoin 20 mg/kg IV
   d. Administer phenobarbital 20 mg/kg IV

Lorazepam should be administered a second time at the same dose. However, at this time you should also begin thinking of additional therapeutic measures. For any patient outside of the neonatal period, phenytoin is the most appropriate next step in management. Fosphenytoin, the water soluble prodrug of phenytoin, has been touted because it does not contain propylene glycol necessary to make phenytoin water soluble. Propylene glycol causes hypotension and therefore phenytoin must be administered over 30 minutes, whereas fosphenytoin can be administered rapidly. The onset of action of both is about 30 to 60 minutes, so the benefit of rapid administration has been questioned. A real benefit of fosphenytoin is that it lacks the tissue toxicity of phenytoin and is less sclerosing to veins. A major disadvantage of fosphenytoin is its price, many times that of phenytoin.

7. Several minutes following his second dose of lorazepam, the patient develops shallow breathing, while continuing to seize. What is your next step?
   a. Administer fosphenytoin 20 mg/kg IV
   b. Place an oral airway
   c. Prepare for immediate intubation
   d. Obtain STAT head CT

Airway management is necessary for patients with prolonged seizure and in those who are not maintaining airway patency. An oral airway is often difficult to place in a patient who is seizing, and furthermore it may lead to vomiting and aspiration. A nasopharyngeal airway, which does not induce gagging, is a great airway adjunct in seizure that will allow sufficient patency for oxygenation. Intubation is often necessary in prolonged seizure where multiple doses of benzodiazepine are required. You intubate successfully and next administer fosphenytoin. Five minutes later his seizure activity stops. A head CT is done which is normal. He is transferred to the pediatric intensive care unit (PICU) for EEG monitoring and a neurological evaluation.

Answers: 1-e, 2-c, 3-a, 4-e, 5-d, 6-a, 7-c

DEFINITION

A *seizure* results when there is an excessive and abnormal discharge of activity from cortical neurons. Symptoms can include impairment or loss of consciousness, abnormal motor activity, abnormal behavior, abnormal sensation, or autonomic dysfunction. A *generalized seizure* involves loss of consciousness and can be subdivided into several subtypes based on the phenotype of the seizure activity. These subtypes include absence, atonic, tonic-clonic, tonic, myoclonic, or infantile spasms. *Partial* (also referred to as *focal*) seizures are defined as those in which consciousness is preserved and *complex partial* seizures are those in which consciousness is impaired. *Epilepsy* refers to at least two unprovoked seizures separated by at least 1 day in time. *Status epilepticus* is technically defined as three or more sequential seizures without full recovery of consciousness between seizures, or more than 30 minutes of continuous seizure activity. There are many physicians, however, who consider any patient with persistent witnessed seizure activity for greater than 5 minutes, intermittent clinical seizures for at least 15 minutes, or continuous electroencephalographic seizures for at least 15 minutes to clinically be in status epilepticus.

What Is NOT a Seizure?

There are several disorders that may be mistaken for seizures and that should therefore be considered in the differential diagnosis of seizure disorders.

Syncope presents with a sudden and transient loss of consciousness and muscle tone. However, syncopal events, unlike seizures, are typically preceded by a sensation of light-headedness, dizziness, nausea, or vomiting. Breath-holding spells occur in up to 5% of healthy children and are typified by a characteristic sequence of events like crying, noiseless expiration, color change to pale or cyanotic, loss of consciousness, and postural tone. Occasionally, there may even be urinary incontinence and movements similar to myoclonic jerks. These events usually occur by 2 years of age and in more than half the cases will disappear by age 4 and nearly all by age 8.

Migraine headaches can be preceded by an aura, motor dysfunction, or clouded consciousness and therefore may be confused with a seizure disorder, particularly in patients with complicated migraine who have associated transient hemiparesis. A normal level of consciousness can distinguish the two, as can the duration of symptoms as migraines typically have a much longer duration than seizures. Paresthesias and visual phenomena related to migraine headaches tend to be of longer duration than those associated with seizures arising from either the parietal or occipital lobes, respectively.

Apparent life-threatening events (ALTEs) often present with symptoms that can easily be confused with seizures in young infants. Symptoms may include choking, gagging, apnea, cyanosis, and/or abnormal muscle tone. In fact, up to one-third of children admitted to the hospital to undergo diagnostic evaluation for an ALTE will be diagnosed with seizure.

Pseudoseizures occur most often in teenage girls with a previously diagnosed seizure disorder and typically consist of bilateral thrashing activity. Pseudoseizures can be difficult to distinguish from a true seizure disorder, although it is noteworthy that patients with pseudoseizures rarely injure themselves even in the setting of their typically violent seizure activity. Sleep disorders such as, night terrors and nightmares, can also be confused with seizure disorders and therefore should be considered in the differential diagnosis.

Gather Clues while Performing the History and Physical Examination

Any possible precipitating factors should be elicited while obtaining the history from the patient, caregiver, and any available witnesses. Questions should specifically seek any possible exposures such as toxins or medications, any trauma (accidental or nonaccidental) and any history of fever in the recent past or present. A thorough prior medical history and family history may also contribute to the diagnosis. If possi-

LITERATURE REFERENCE

ALTE: A seizure mimicker

ALTEs are episodes characterized by some combination of events, which in the caregiver's eyes place the child at risk for death. Most episodes contain apnea or breathing irregularities, color changes, choking, gagging, and/or changes in mental status or muscle tone. Most infants appear normal by the time they present to the emergency department. Brand et al. performed an observational study in which they reviewed the records of 243 patients who carried a diagnosis of ALTE to determine the yield of different diagnostic tests in helping to identify the etiology. The top three final diagnoses in their study were gastroesophageal reflux, bronchiolitis, and afebrile seizures. They specifically analyzed the subgroup of patients with a nonsuggestive history and normal physical examination and found that the only tests which had a significant yield when performed on this subgroup were gastroesophageal reflux screening, urine analysis and culture, brain neuroimaging, pneumogram, and white blood cell count. Broad evaluations for systemic infections, metabolic diseases, and blood chemistry abnormalities were not found to be productive in this subgroup. Nevertheless, these guidelines have not yet been accepted into common practice and the need to supplement the above short list with additional testing should be individualized and dictated by clinical judgment [Brand DA et al. *Pediatrics.* 2005;115(4)885–893].

ble, obtaining a detailed description of the event can provide vital information as well. Key information involves defining any precipitating events or focality to the seizure, its duration, and identifying any change in the patient's level of consciousness. Physical examination findings can also help in determining the etiology (see Box 11-1).

How Much Diagnostic Evaluation Is Enough but Not Too Much?

Routine laboratory investigation is not necessarily indicated in a child over 6 months of age with a history of seizure disorder, unless there is a suspicion for toxic ingestion or underlying illness that may lead to

The physical examination is also used to identify a possible etiology for the seizure. A reliable temperature should be obtained as part of a complete set of vital signs. The head should be examined for evidence of trauma. Pupil size and reactivity, extraocular eye muscle movements, and optic disc margins should be carefully evaluated. The presence of retinal hemorrhages strongly support nonaccidental trauma and should not be missed. The elicitation of meningeal signs should be attempted, particularly in febrile children, although their absence in children less than 18 months should not be considered definitive. A thorough examination of the skin should note the presence of any rashes, pigmented or hypopigmented lesions or anything else suggestive of a neurocutaneous syndrome. Finally, a detailed neurologic examination should be performed including an accurate assessment of a patient's mental status. If a patient appears postictal during any phase of the evaluation, then a return to baseline mental status should be followed.

Metabolic
  Lactic acidosis
  Hypercapnia
  Hyperkalemia
  Hyponatremia
  Hypoglycemia
  Serum leukocytosis

Autonomic
  Hyperpyrexia
  Vomiting
  Incontinence
  Cerebral autoregulation failure

Cardiac
  Arrhythmia
  High output failure

Respiratory
  Pneumonia
  Hypoxia

Renal
  Myoglobinuria
  Rhabdomyolysis
  Acute renal failure (ARF)

electrolyte disturbances. A fingerstick glucose should be checked in diabetic children or simply administer glucose IV or glucagon intramuscularly (IM) if actively seizing. Any child less than 6 months of age should have blood drawn for electrolytes, calcium, and magnesium. Hypocalcemia and hyponatremia are associated with seizures (see Box 11-2). For infants who are less than 1 month old, the differential diagnosis is much broader and therefore necessitates a more extensive evaluation. This topic is further discussed below.

Routine head imaging is not indicated in the evaluation of a first nonfebrile seizure in children. However, head imaging should be strongly considered in any patient with any of the following risk factors: head trauma, focal seizure activity, seizure duration greater than 15 minutes, focal postictal deficits that do not rapidly resolve, or persistent altered level of consciousness. Similarly, children with a medical history that places them at risk for intracranial events should also be evaluated with appropriate neuroimaging. Several specific conditions include sickle cell disease (increased risk for stroke), bleeding disorders (increased risk for hemorrhage and/or stroke) malignancy (increased risk for mass lesion and/or stroke), and human immunodeficiency virus (HIV) (increased risk for opportunistic infections). Specifically, magnetic resonance imaging (MRI) should be considered in any patient less than 1 year, particularly with delayed developmental milestones, as well as in any patient with focal seizure activity or persistent neurologic abnormalities on examination.

EEG analysis is indicated in the evaluation of any first-time seizure. However, typically this study does not need to be obtained on an emergent basis and is often coordinated as outpatient care. In fact, if the EEG is performed within the first 24 to 48 hours following a seizure, it can have postictal slowing and that may limit its prognostic ability. An emergent EEG is helpful in children who fail to return to baseline mental status following seizure activity. EEG is also necessary in patients who are intubated and sedated in order to control the seizure; these patients may still have neuronal discharge despite the lack of muscle contraction.

TREATMENT

Initial management of seizure should start with airway, breathing, and safety. Supplemental oxygen should always be provided, preferably via a 100% nonrebreather mask. A nasopharyngeal airway can be quite helpful for maintaining airway patency; suctioning may also be helpful to clear secretion and prevent aspiration. Typically breathing, although altered and often disturbing to an onlooker, remains effective until suppressed by pharmacotherapy administration. A quick pulse check should be done and the patient attached to a monitor. If the child is diabetic, fingerstick glucose should be checked. If there is delay or hypoglycemia (less than 40 mg/dL), 2 to 4 mL/kg of D25W should be administered as a bolus. For patients less than 1 month old, 2 to 4 mL/kg of D10W should be used.

Pharmacotherapy is indicated in any child who has a seizure which lasts greater than 5 minutes, as does any child who presents to the ED actively seizing (i.e., unclear but prolonged duration). Benzodiazepines are the initial antiepileptic drug of choice. Lorazepam (Ativan) is preferred due to its longer duration of action and the recommended dose is 0.1 mg/kg IV. If IV access is not obtained, then rectal administration of diazepam (Valium) is indicated at a dose of 0.5 mg/kg. Both of these drugs typically have an onset of action within 2 to 3 minutes but can take up to 5 minutes.

If seizure activity persists 5 minutes beyond the initial administration of either lorazepam or diazepam, then a second round of either of these drugs at the same dose is indicated. It is essential to continually monitor the effectiveness of the patient's breathing as benzodiazepines suppress the respiratory drive, therefore further compromising an already compromised system. Intubation should be performed immediately whenever there is concern for ineffective oxygenation and ventilation.

Additional classes of antiepileptic agents should be utilized for seizures, which continue despite two rounds of benzodiazepine administration. Phenytoin 20 mg/kg IV over 30 minutes, or its prodrug fosphenytoin 20 mg/kg IV bolus, should be administered next in patients greater than 1 year of age. Fosphenytoin, if available, is preferred due to its decreased risk profile and ease of administration, although it is very expensive. Both these drugs have a delayed onset of action, typically 30 to 45 minutes. Phenobarbital 20 mg/kg IV/IM is typically used in patients less than 1 year of age, although phenytoin and fosphenytoin are gaining acceptance in this younger age group as well (see Table 11-1).

When It Just Doesn't Break

Induction of deep sedation is required in status epilepticus refractory to the above treatments. This requires endotracheal intubation, preferably done with rapid sequence intubation (RSI). Pentobarbital induces a profound depression in consciousness and respiratory drive, resulting in what is referred to as a "barbiturate coma." Pentobarbital had previously been the drug of choice for refractory seizures, although it is a potent negative inotrope and can result in hypotension. Propofol, though also a negative inotrope, is probably more commonly used in this scenario today. Even though pentobarbital and propofol render the patient unconscious, neuronal discharge can take place with-

TABLE 11-1 Know your meds!				
Medication	**Loading dose**	**Rate of administration**	**Onset of action**	**Side effect**
Lorazepam (Ativan)	0.1 mg/kg IV (max dose 4 mg)	Slowly over 1 to 2 min	3 to 5 min	Respiratory, depression, hypotension, sialorrhea
Diazepam (Valium)	0.1 to 0.3 mg/kg IV (max dose 10 mg) 0.5 mg/kg [S1]PR (max dose 20 mg)	Slow IV push	1 to 2 min	
Midazolam (Versed)	0.3 mg/kg IM		1 to 2 min	Respiratory, depression, hypotension
Phenytoin (Dilantin)	20 mg/kg IV	<1 mg/kg/min	10 to 30 min	Cardiac depression, hypotension
Fosphenytoin	20 mg PE/kg IV	3 mg PE/kg/min	15 to 30 min	
Phenobarbital	20 mg/kg IV/IM	<1 mg/kg/min	20 to 60 min	Respiratory depression, bradycardia, hypotension
Pentobarbital	5 to 10 mg/kg IV	<1 mg/kg/min	1 min	Hypotension
Propofol	1 to 3 mg/kg/h IV	1 to 2 mg/kg/min	1 min	Bradycardia, apnea, hypotension
Valproic acid	15 to 20 mg/kg IV		6 to 10 min	None significant

out motor seizure activity itself. Therefore, patients who receive pentobarbital must also have continuous EEG monitoring in an ICU setting.

Further Workup

Patients with a history of seizure disorder who seize for 2 to 3 minutes followed by a postictal period of 10 to 15 minutes can simply be observed without any further workup. Drug levels (e.g., phenytoin, valproic acid) should be checked and repleted if low. A reason for the acute seizure should be sought, whether it is noncompliance with dosing, recent infection, lack of sleep, or use of stimulants. Patients require admission for prolonged seizures (i.e., greater than 20 minutes) or increased seizure frequency while compliant with medications. Patients also warrant admission if the etiology of seizure is thought due to something other than epilepsy (e.g., electrolyte disturbances, toxic ingestions, infection, head trauma). These patients require further monitoring and management to ensure the underlying cause is addressed.

Fever Is a Special Consideration

Febrile seizures are defined as seizures which occur in the setting of fever but without evidence for an intracranial infection and in the absence of any known seizure disorder. They are the most common convulsive disorder of childhood. It is estimated that between 3% and 5% of children aged 6 months to 5 years will experience a febrile seizure, with the median age of onset between 17 and 23 months of life. This occurrence rate is increased in families where there is a history of childhood febrile seizures. The recurrence risk for a second febrile seizure is roughly 30% and the risk for a third climbs to 50%. Typically, febrile seizures occur within the first 24 hours of illness, and actually up to 50% of patients will have a seizure as their first sign of a febrile illness, as seizures are more related to sudden changes in temperature rather than to the absolute height of a fever. Having said that, it is also important to warn that the mean fever in patients with febrile seizures is quite high (39.8°C), but this has not been found to be associated with an increased rate of serious bacterial illness beyond the general population risk.

    The most important branch point in the management of patients with febrile seizures involves the classification of the seizure as either simple or complex. Most (80%) of all febrile seizures are simple, meaning that they are generalized, last less than 15 minutes and

LITERATURE REFERENCE

The heat is rising! A look at the evaluation of simple febrile seizures

Simple febrile seizures are defined as primary generalized seizures lasting ≤15 minutes and not recurring within 24 hours. Complex febrile seizures are defined as focal, prolonged (>15 minutes), and/or occurring in a flurry with multiple seizure episodes within 24 hours. The most recent practice parameter released by the American Academy of Pediatrics (AAP) in 1996 suggests that an LP should be done on children less than one year of age and strongly considered in those 12 to 18 months of age or those who have received prior antibiotics. In each of these groups, clinical signs of meningitis may be absent or subtle. After 18 months, clinical signs are more reliable. The following are not routinely recommended: blood work, neuroimaging, or EEG [Bergman DA et al. *Pediatrics.* 1996;97:769–772].

occur only once within a 24-hour period. Simple febrile seizures carry few risks of complications and have excellent short and long-term prognoses. These children do not require a diagnostic workup if they do not have any evidence of intracranial infection on examination and if they are greater than 1 year of age.

    A febrile seizure is considered complex when it has focal features, lasts for more than 15 minutes, or if seizure activity occurs more than once in a 24-hour period. Complex febrile seizures require more extensive evaluation. The workup should include serum electrolytes, head CT, LP, and outpatient EEG. Patients with a complex febrile seizure have a 6% incidence of developing epilepsy later in life. In contrast, simple febrile seizures carry a 1% incidence of epilepsy later in life, twice the incidence of the general population.

Beware of Seizures in the Very Young

Neonatal seizures typically occur within the first week of life and are often less obvious than seizure activity in older children and adults. Typically neonatal seizures are identified by unusual repetitive and stereotypic movements and often have multifocality, asynchrony of clonic activity, and a lack of generalized tonic-clonic activity. Similarly, in contrast to seizures in older children, neonatal seizures are much less often idiopathic and instead can be traced to one of several etiologies including intracranial hemorrhage, metabolic derangements such as inborn errors of metabolism, hyponatremia or hypoglycemia, intracranial infection, and cerebral structural anomalies.

KEY POINTS

- First-time seizure in child >6 months does not require workup
  - Exception if suspicion for specific etiology
  - Outpatient EEG indicated
- Think of abuse
  - Look for retinal hemorrhages or external evidence of trauma
- Address ABCs and safety first in seizure
  - Nasopharyngeal airway and supplemental oxygen
- Benzodiazepines are first-line therapy
  - Lorazepam (Ativan) or diazepam (Valium)
- Phenytoin/fosphenytoin is second-line therapy for persistent seizure
- Refractory seizures require pentobarbital, midazolam, propofol, or valproic acid
- Never miss hypoglycemia!
  - Fingerstick glucose in diabetics or patient without a known seizure disorder
- LP should be strongly considered in simple febrile seizure in those <18 months
- Complex febrile seizures are uncommon and require an extensive evaluation
- Neonatal seizures often present without generalized tonic-clonic seizure activity and instead with stereotypic and repetitive movements
  - EEG, head imaging, LP, and extensive laboratory work is indicated
  - Suspect structural anomalies, inborn errors of metabolism, infection, and electrolyte abnormalities

CHAPTER 12

Anaphylaxis

CASE SCENARIO

A 6-year-old boy is brought to the ED by ambulance for a suspected episode of anaphylaxis following a meal at a local Chinese food restaurant approximately 15 minutes prior to arrival to the ED. His parents report that he developed flushing and itching within 5 minutes of starting his meal. He then developed hives and started to complain of difficulty breathing. En route to the ED, he received an albuterol nebulizer. He arrives by stretcher with an oxygen mask on his face.

1. Which of the following factors is associated with severe food allergic reactions?
    a. Male gender
    b. History of poorly controlled asthma
    c. Age 6 years
    d. Tachycardia

Age in and of itself does not predict severity of reaction. It is, however, predictive of the type of reagent that produces the anaphylactic response. Adults are more prone to reactions to certain drugs and Hymenoptera stings (bees and wasps), while children are much more likely to develop allergic reactions to food. Both genders are affected equally in children. Tachycardia is a hallmark sign of anaphylaxis and not predictive of severity of reaction. Prior history of atopy is associated with a higher fatality rate, particularly in children with daily symptoms of asthma.

Further questioning of this patient's family reveals that he has had three prior hospitalizations for asthma and that he uses his albuterol inhaler roughly three times per day. Budesonide (Pulmicort) has been prescribed for him in the past; however, his parents inform you that they do not reliably administer this medication. He has not had any prior episodes of anaphylaxis and they are not aware of any food or drug allergies.

His vital signs on arrival include a pulse of 140, blood pressure 75/45, respiratory rate 46, and arterial oxygen concentration (SaO_2) 100% nonrebreather (NRB) mask 99%. His weight is approximately 30 kg. He is awake but in moderate respiratory distress. His head, eyes, ears, nose, and throat (HEENT) examination reveals no evidence of upper airway edema. His skin examination reveals flushing and diffuse hives. Auscultation of his chest reveals diffuse wheezes with moderate air exchange. He has mild subcostal and suprasternal retractions. He has no stridor.

2. What is the next best step in his management?
    a. Administer epinephrine 0.3 mg intramuscularly (IM)
    b. Prepare for intubation
    c. Administer 20 cc/kg normal saline (NS) bolus
    d. Administer albuterol 2.5 mg via nebulizer

Protecting the airway is your first priority. An argument can be made to intubate this child immediately given his moderate respiratory distress and retractions. This may be wise as there is yet no evidence of upper airway edema. Once the airway becomes edematous, it may be impossible to intubate the child. An oxygen saturation of 100% should not be reassuring as children often compensate adequately until respiratory failure ensues. It is reasonable at this point to administer epinephrine, as its effect is usually very rapid. Epinephrine is the drug of choice for anaphylaxis because it can reverse both bronchospasm and hypotension. Aqueous epinephrine 1:1,000 dilution should be administered *intramuscularly* at a dose of 0.01 mg/kg in children with a maximum one-time dosage of 0.3 mg. It can be administered at intervals of 5 minutes until symptoms have improved with an upper limit of three doses.

While epinephrine administration should be your first priority with this patient, intravenous IV access must also be established for fluid administration. His blood pressure is low for his age (normal systolic blood pressure (SBP) >82 for 6-year-old) and may continue to fall as fluid shifts from the intravascular to extravascular space. This is a result of increased vascular permeability induced by massive histamine release. He should receive an NS bolus of 20 cc/kg. This can be repeated several times to a rough maximum dosage of 60 cc/kg; but if hypotension persists despite IM epinephrine and multiple fluid boluses, additional vasopressor support should be considered, such as IV epinephrine or dopamine. Nebulized albuterol is another option for managing bronchospasm in the setting of anaphylaxis, particularly in children with a history of asthma. However, albuterol administration should only be provided in conjunction with epinephrine administration and should never be used as an isolated therapy when anaphylaxis is suspected.

You administer a dose of IM epinephrine and then place an IV to deliver a 20 cc/kg NS bolus. Within minutes he reports that his breathing feels better and following administration of the fluid bolus his SBP has improved to 85 mm/Hg.

3. What is the next best step in his management?
   a. Administer diphenhydramine 1 mg/kg IV
   b. Administer ranitidine 1 mg/kg IV
   c. Administer epinephrine (1:10,000) 0.01 mg/kg IV epinephrine
   d. Administer Solu-Medrol (methyl-prednisolone sodium succinate) 2 mg/kg IV
   e. Both a and b

While epinephrine is considered first-line therapy for anaphylaxis, H_1 and H_2 blockers such as diphenhydramine and ranitidine, respectively, also play important roles in the management of anaphylaxis. The combination of both has been shown to be superior to either independently and these should be administered early in the course of treatment following appropriate epinephrine therapy. Systemic glucocorticoids are essential for patients with anaphylaxis, particularly in those who have a history of asthma or who have had severe and prolonged anaphylactic symptoms. Steroids blunt the secondary inflammatory response that includes leukocyte migration, leukotriene and prostaglandin release, and resulting airway inflammation and edema. The steroid effect is not immediate, but it prevents recurrence of symptoms after the first-line agents for the allergic reaction have worn off.

Anaphylaxis is a clinical diagnosis and prompt treatment is necessary based on symptoms and signs; however, laboratory confirmation may be helpful in the diagnostic process if the history is unclear.

4. Which laboratory test would be most helpful to confirm the diagnosis of anaphylaxis?
   a. Rapid antigen serum testing (RAST)
   b. Skin testing
   c. Serum tryptase levels
   d. Plasma histamine levels

RAST and skin testing are considered the most useful diagnostic tests for food allergy, but they do not confirm the diagnosis of anaphylaxis. RAST testing can be performed in the immediate period surrounding a presumed anaphylactic episode and may be helpful; however, the specificity is low (roughly 50%) and may be misleading. Skin testing is more specific, but should be delayed at least 6 weeks following an acute episode of allergy. Serum tryptase is a protease specific to mast cells. When it is elevated, it is considered to be strong evidence for mast cell degranulation, which is the primary pathophysiology of anaphylaxis. Therefore, the measurement of serum tryptase can be a very helpful diagnostic test if the etiology of a child's respiratory distress is unclear. Because tryptase levels peak 60 to 90 minutes following the onset of anaphylaxis and persist for only up to 6 hours, the level must typically be obtained in the ED and will not be useful if obtained more than 6 hours following the development of symptoms. Plasma histamine levels can also be helpful in establishing the diagnosis; however, they are often difficult to obtain due to their rapid clearance. Histamine levels rise within 10 minutes of exposure and remain increased for only 30 to 60 minutes.

Within 2 hours the patient is feeling back to near baseline with only several hives remaining on examination. His parents are requesting to go home.

5. What is the best disposition for this patient?
   a. Home with primary care physician (PCP) follow-up the next day
   b. Home with allergy/immunology follow-up the next day
   c. Observation in the ED for 2 more hours, then home if stable
   d. Admission for continued observation

Biphasic reactions are seen in up to 20% of patients. Thus, a recurrence of symptoms could occur for up to roughly 8 hours following the patient's initial episode. Biphasic reactions are more common in patients who have been exposed to the antigen via the oral route or in patients who developed initial symptoms greater than 30 minutes following exposure. Thus, the patient in this scenario with a suspected food allergy is at risk for a biphasic reaction and should be admitted for observation.

Answers: 1-b, 2-a, 3-e, 4-c, 5-d

Who, What, Where and Why?

The term anaphylaxis is derived from the Greek words *ana* (against) and *phylaxis* (immunity, protection). There is currently no universally accepted clinical definition of anaphylaxis. Some clinicians define it broadly as a syndrome of one or more systemic signs and symptoms, whereas others require either dyspnea or hypotension to make the diagnosis. In general, however, anaphylaxis refers to the potentially life-threatening symptoms which result from immunoglobulin E (IgE) mediated immediate hypersensitivity reactions (see Table 12-1). *Anaphylactoid* reactions present with clinical signs and symptoms identical to those seen in anaphylaxis, but they are not immune mediated (see Box 12-1).

The estimated risk of anaphylaxis per person in the United States is 1% to 3%. Approximately 1,000 deaths from anaphylaxis occur in the United States each year, equaling a mortality rate of roughly 1%. Adults are more prone to anaphylactic reactions to medications, most commonly penicillin. They also have a higher incidence of reactions to Hymenoptera stings, radiocontrast media, and anesthetic agents. Children, on the other hand, most commonly have allergic reactions to food. Girls and boys have a similar incidence of anaphylaxis to most antigens. Atopic individuals appear to have an increased risk of experiencing an anaphylactic reaction to multiple exposures including food. Those atopic individuals with poorly controlled asthma are at increased risk for severe anaphylactic reactions and death, and patients with a previous history of severe type 1 immediate hypersensitivity reactions are also at increased risk for anaphylaxis.

TABLE 12-1 Classifying allergic reactions

Type 1	Immediate-type hypersensitivity	Occurs when antigens attach to specific IgE antibody on mast cells or basophils causing them to release vasoactive substances such as histamine, prostaglandins, and leukotrienes. Examples include anaphylaxis, urticaria, bronchospasm, and angioedema.
Type 2	Antibody-dependent cytotoxicity	Occurs when an antigen that is immediately related to a cell binds to either IgG or IgM antibody with subsequent complement fixation leading to cell death. An example is hemolytic anemia.
Type 3	Immune complex disease	Occurs when antigen-antibody complexes deposit in blood vessels or tissue with subsequent complement fixation. An example is serum sickness.
Type 4	Cell-mediated or delayed hypersensitivity	Occurs when an antigen exposure sensitizes T cells, which subsequently mediate tissue injury. No antibody is involved. Examples include contact dermatitis and tuberculin-type hypersensitivity.

IgE, immunoglobulin E; IgG, immunoglobulin G; IgM, immunoglobulin M.

- Hereditary angioedema
- Asthma
- Systemic mast cell disorders
- Acute poisoning
- Foreign body aspiration
- Hypoglycemia
- Seizure disorder
- Myocardial dysfunction
- Pulmonary embolism
- Vasovagal reactions
- Acute anxiety

Anaphylaxis occurs when a patient is exposed to an antigen that activates IgE to bind to mast cells and basophils. This leads to the release of preformed vasoactive substances including histamine, prostaglandins, leukotrienes, platelet activating factor, and tryptase. These mediators induce a number of systemic responses including increased vascular permeability, vasodilation, respiratory smooth muscle contraction, autonomic nervous system stimulation, mucous secretion, platelet aggregation, and recruitment of inflammatory cells. These physiologic changes then lead to the constellation of symptoms associated with anaphylaxis. The most common symptoms seen in anaphylaxis are urticaria and angioedema. In fact, at least 90% of patients with anaphylaxis experience at least one of these two symptoms.

It is important to note, however, that not all patients with anaphylaxis will have these symptoms. In fact, rapidly progressing anaphylaxis with cardiovascular shock, one of the most severe forms of anaphylaxis, may present without either of these skin findings. Cardiovascular collapse, sometimes referred to as anaphylactic shock, occurs in up to 30% of patients and results from the loss of up to 50% of circulating blood volume to the extravascular space due to the tremendous increase in vascular permeability. Respiratory tract involvement, typically characterized by complaints of shortness of breath with wheezing on examination, occurs in roughly 50% of patients. Gastrointestinal (GI) symptoms, typically nausea, abdominal cramping, or diarrhea, occur in approximately 30% of patients.

Act Fast with Epinephrine!

The treatment for all patients with symptoms consistent with anaphylaxis is the immediate delivery of epinephrine as it has the ability to counteract both bronchoconstriction and hypotension. Doses should be memorized so that there is no unnecessary delay: 0.01 mg/kg epinephrine 1:1000 IM or subcutaneous (SC) (maximum dose for each delivery route is 0.3 mg) every 5 minutes as necessary. For patients with critical symptoms such as stridor, severe bronchospasm, or severe hypotension, epinephrine should be administered IM immediately on presentation and switched to IV dosing as vascular access is obtained. A dosage of 0.01 mg/kg (0.1 mL/kg of a 1:10,000 solution) is recommended for children with a maximum IV dose of 0.3 mg. In addition to IV epinephrine, critical patients require aggressive fluid resuscitation due to the massive fluid shifts. Children should be initially resuscitated with 20 cc/kg NS boluses, at least 30 cc/kg within the first hour of resuscitation is often necessary. If IV epinephrine and liberal fluid resuscitation does not achieve hemodynamic stability, then other vasopressor agents such as dopamine should be considered.

Other Common Agents Used in Allergic Reaction

Additional pharmacologic therapy plays a key role in the management of anaphylaxis. Histamine blockers play a very important role in management because they help counteract all of the effects of the vasoactive mediators (as mentioned previously). Studies have shown that both H_1 and H_2 blockers, diphenhydramine (1 mg/kg IV) and ranitidine (1 mg/kg IV), respectively, should be administered to patients with anaphylaxis. Inhaled beta-agonists such as nebulized albuterol should be used in patients with bronchospasm and in all patients with a history of asthma. Systemic glucocorticoids should be given for patients who experience severe allergic reaction or anaphylaxis. If given IV, glucocorticoids should be administered every 6 hours (1 mg/kg/dose). For the rare pediatric patient who is on beta-blockers and who therefore may be resistant to treatment with epinephrine, consider glucagon, which has inotropic and chronotropic effects on the cardiovascular system that are not mediated through beta-receptors.

The Best Medicine Is Prevention (and Preparedness)!

Children who have experienced symptoms consistent with anaphylaxis should be evaluated by an allergist. Skin testing and/or RAST testing should be utilized to help identify a precipitant so that the offending antigen can be avoided. Patients should be educated to use preloaded epinephrine syringes at the first sign of symptoms and to remain in a supine position. The EpiPen contains a dose of epinephrine 0.3 mg and the EpiPen Jr contains 0.15 mg of epinephrine.

LITERATURE REFERENCE

Take it lying down!

Sicherer and Leung recently reviewed and concurred with observations made previously by Humphrey (2000, 2003) that postural changes in patients with anaphylaxis played a significant role in stability. Humphrey noted that in 10 cases of fatal anaphylaxis in which postural information was available that all 10 persons died while in an upright position. In fact, four of the deaths occurred within seconds of the victim being placed upright after being supine. He theorizes that while a person is supine, blood return to the vena cava is sufficient to maintain a reduced circulation. However, venous return decreases even further when a person mobilizes to either a sit or stand position decreasing blood return to the right side of the heart below a critical level which then leads to circulatory collapse and cardiac ischemia. Conversely, patients who remain supine while administering epinephrine and who even raise their legs above the level of their heart may maintain or increase circulation. Therefore for anaphylactic shock, these investigators suggest forgetting the old adage and to instead "take this lying down" **[Sicherer SH et al. _J Allergy Clin Immunol._ 2004;144:118–124]**.

LITERATURE REFERENCE

In a nutshell—IgE antibodies may help prevent anaphylaxis in unintended peanut ingestions

In a double-blind, randomized, dose-ranging trial, Leung et al. investigated the effects of human monoclonal IgE antibody (TNX-901) on 84 patients with known peanut allergies. TNX-901 effectively prevents the binding of peanut antigen to mast cells and basophils by masking the effective epitope. Patients were randomly assigned to receive one of three doses of TNX-901 or placebo subcutaneously every 4 weeks for four doses. The patients underwent a final oral food challenge within 2 to 4 weeks after the fourth dose. They found that a 450-mg dose of TNX-901 significantly and substantially increased the threshold of sensitivity to peanut on oral food challenge from a level equal to approximately half a peanut to the level equal to almost nine peanuts, an effect that should translate into protection against most unintended ingestions of peanuts **[Leung DY et al. _N Emerg J Med._ 2003;348:1046–1048]**.

These items have a limited shelf life of 1 year, a fact that is very important for patients to know. Medic alert bracelets for patients with known allergies are extremely helpful at expediting a diagnosis, especially in children who are often unable to verbalize their history. Human monoclonal antibodies against IgE are currently being evaluated for their potential role in prevention of anaphylaxis and other allergic phenomena.

KEY POINTS

- Anaphylaxis is a type 1 immediate hypersensitivity reaction
  - Antigen-IgE antibody complex on the surface of mast cells
- Anaphylactoid reactions similar clinically to anaphylaxis
  - Not mediated by IgE
- Symptoms are multisystem
  - Airway—laryngeal edema and stridor; bronchospasm and wheeze
  - Cutaneous—urticaria
    - Not always present in anaphylaxis
  - GI—cramps, vomiting, diarrhea
  - Vascular— vasodilation, hypotension
- Anaphylaxis often produces signs within minutes of exposure
  - Late-phase reaction may occur up to 12 hours out
- Treatment
  - Epinephrine 1:1,000 (0.01 mg/kg, max 0.3 mg) IM every 5 minutes as needed
  - Aggressive fluid resuscitation for hypotension and shock
  - Histamine blockers (H_1 and H_2)
  - Inhaled bronchodilators (beta-agonists)
  - Glucocorticoids to prevent late-phase reaction
- Serum tryptase level can be helpful within first 6 hours if diagnosis in question

CHAPTER 13

Croup

CASE SCENARIO

A 20-month-old boy is brought to the ED at 2 a.m. with a chief complaint of cough. His mother states that he has had a runny nose, cough, and fever over the past 2 days. She put him down to bed at 8 p.m. but his cough has been getting worse throughout the night and keeps waking him from sleep. She describes the cough as dry and sounds very hoarse. He has been agitated, but his cough has improved since going outside and coming to the hospital. His vitals reveal a temperature of 39°C, heart rate of 120, respiratory rate of 34, and pulse oximetry of 94%. His physical examination reveals inspiratory stridor while crying during the examination with moderate accessory muscle use and retractions, as well as a loud, dry cough.

1. What is the most likely cause of his stridor?
   a. Foreign body
   b. Subglottic edema
   c. Epiglottitis
   d. Vascular ring

In patients with inspiratory stridor, it is important to rule out serious infection such as epiglottitis. Children with epiglottitis are typically toxic appearing, drooling, and refuse to lie supine. A foreign body in either the airway or esophagus may decrease airflow and usually is acute in onset. A vascular ring may cause chronic stridor from persistent tracheal compression. Our patient most likely has croup, which is characterized by subglottic edema, which causes a hoarse cough often referred to as a "barking cough."

2. Which of the following treatments is indicated for this patient?
   a. Humidified oxygen
   b. Racemic epinephrine nebulizer treatment
   c. Steroids
   d. All of the above

Patients with croup benefit from humidified oxygen as it helps clear respiratory secretions and makes them feel comfortable. Epinephrine given via a nebulizer causes arteriole vasoconstriction and a reduction in subglottic edema, which improves respiratory distress. Steroids are also proven to decrease inflammation and edema that contributes to respiratory distress. The patient is given blow-by oxygen as a racemic epinephrine nebulizer is prepared. Dexamethasone 0.6 mg/kg is given by mouth. An hour after his epinephrine nebulizer the patient is considerably more comfortable with minimal retractions, good air entry, and an oxygen saturation of 98%. He is drinking apple juice and playing with his mom.

3. Which is the most appropriate next step?
   a. Discharge home
   b. Admit for further epinephrine treatment
   c. Observation in ED for 2 more hours
   d. Chest x-ray and complete blood count (CBC)

Most patients with croup can be managed at home. The duration of effect of an epinephrine nebulizer treatment is about 2 hours. When this wears off, arterioles dilate and swelling can recur, the so-called rebound phenomenon. Patients can be discharged home if they are breathing comfortably and without stridor, if they do not require oxygen to maintain oxygen saturations above 95%, and if they can tolerate liquids. The classic radiographic finding in croup is the "steeple sign," which refers to the trachea as it narrows to a point inferior to the vocal cords. However, there is no need for routine radiographs in croup unless the diagnosis is uncertain or if pneumonia is suspected. Similarly, a CBC is not typically indicated.

The child continues to do well and is observed for a total of 3 hours after the epinephrine nebulizer treatment. He is sleeping comfortably with oxygen saturation above 97%, and he has no retractions. He is sent home and instructed to return to the ED if his stridor worsens.

Answers: 1-b, 2-d, 3-c

DEFINITION

Croup, or laryngotracheobronchitis, is a viral infection of the upper respiratory tract characterized by inspiratory stridor, cough, hoarseness, and fever. A dry, barking "seal-like" cough is the hallmark of the disease. Croup mainly affects young children with small airways, with a peak incidence at 18 months. It is more common in males and recurrence is common, although it rarely affects children older than 6 years of age. Symptoms are typically worse at night and may awaken the child from sleep. Scoring systems have been developed that help characterize disease severity; typically they characterize level of consciousness, presence of cyanosis and stridor at rest or with agitation, and the amount of air entry and retractions (see Box 13-1). The disease is most often mild and self-limited but may progress to significant airway obstruction and rarely death.

BOX 13-1 Differential diagnosis of stridor

- Croup
- Epiglottitis
- Tracheitis
- Retropharyngeal abscess
- Anaphylaxis
- Foreign body
- Nasal deformities
- Macroglossia
- Laryngomalacia
- Laryngeal webs/cysts
- Subglottic hemangioma
- Subglottic stenosis
- Tracheal stenosis
- Vascular ring
- Tracheomalacia
- Vocal cord paralysis

ETIOLOGY

Croup is caused by viruses. The most common is parainfluenza type 1, although other parainfluenza strains, respiratory syncytial virus, adenovirus, and influenza are also frequent causes. The virus typically has a prodrome of nasal congestion and fever. As infection spreads to the larynx and trachea, edema causes swelling and narrowing of the airway in the subglottic region. An inflammatory exudate also contributes to a compromised upper airway. Air flowing through the narrowed airway causes the high-pitched inspiratory noise known as stridor.

MANAGEMENT

With aggressive ED management few cases of croup require hospitalization. The degree of intervention is dependent on the degree of respiratory distress. Those with hypoxia, stridor at rest, significant work of breathing, or obtundation require immediate treatment.

CLINICAL PEARL

Parainfluenza, an odd virus

Parainfluenza virus is the most common cause of croup. It also has a very unique epidemiology. Parainfluenza 1 causes large biennial outbreaks of croup in the fall and winter of odd-numbered years. Outbreaks of parainfluenza 2 commonly follow parainfluenza 1 outbreaks. Parainfluenza 3 in contrast appears yearly, but mainly in spring and summer. Since parainfluenza 1 is by far the most common cause of croup, EDs are usually much busier with croup in the fall of odd-numbered years.

Airway and Breathing

Evaluate the adequacy of the airway for effective oxygenation and ventilation. Oxygen should be given for any child who is hypoxemic or in respiratory distress. Intubation is rarely needed but if necessary for maintenance of airway patency, an endotracheal tube 0.5 to 1 mm smaller than predicted should be used to account for the swollen airway. While monitoring of the heart rate, respiratory rate, and pulse oximetry are important to detect hypoxia in severe illness, it may be best to avoid these interventions in mild disease. Agitation and crying increase oxygen demands and may worsen symptoms.

Humidity—Cool and Wet Is How They Like It

Humidified air has long been a treatment of croup although there are few studies that verify its efficacy. The water droplets in the air decrease the viscosity of tracheal secretions, which facilitates clearance. All oxygen given should be humidified. This can be accomplished through nebulizers with saline, blow-by, or through oxygen mist tents. At home, parents can sit the patient in the bathroom with a hot shower running. Cool mist may also be helpful, as parents often report bringing the patient into the cold night air improves symptoms. This may be an effect of cold-induced vasoconstriction of the upper airways, lessening the subglottic edema.

Epinephrine to Squeeze Out the Edema

Nebulized epinephrine results in rapid improvement of symptoms in croup. Constriction of arterioles in the upper airway leads to increased fluid resorption and improvement of airway edema. The effect usually takes about 30 minutes and lasts about 2 hours. There is no difference between racemic epinephrine and

TABLE 13-1 Doses of epinephrine for nebulization

Medication	Dose	Max dose
Racemic epinephrine 2.25% solution	0.05 mL/kg diluted in 3 mL normal saline (NS)	0.5 mL
L-epinephrine 1:1,000 solution	0.5 mL/kg diluted in 3 mL NS	<4 yr: 2.5 mL >4 yr: 5 mL

Rebound phenomenon

Rebound effect is a misnomer in that it actually refers to the drug wearing off, not an actual worsening of symptoms. In the past, children who received epinephrine nebulizers in the ED were admitted for observation due to fear of the rebound effect. Multiple studies have proven that it is safe to send children home after nebulized epinephrine if the following criteria are met: no stridor at rest, normal work of breathing, and normal level of consciousness after a period of observation in the ED [Rizos JD. et al. *J Emerg Med.*1998;16:535–539].

standard epinephrine as far as efficacy and side effects are concerned (see Table 13-1). Nebulizers should be given over 15 minutes and may be repeated up to three times. Patients should be placed on a cardiac monitor to observe for arrhythmias. The rebound phenomenon (improvement followed by

Seals on steroids: Should all children with croup be given steroids?

Steroids are the mainstay of treatment for severe and moderate croup. Additionally, steroids in mild disease (barking cough, no stridor at rest, and no respiratory distress) have a significant improvement on the course of the disease. In a multicenter trial of 720 children randomly assigned to a single oral dose of either dexamethasone 0.6 mg/kg or placebo, the steroid-treated group was associated with decreased return visits to medical care, more rapid resolution of symptoms, more sleep for the patient, and less parental stress. It appears steroids should be given for all patients presenting with croup [Bjornson CL et al. *N Engl J Med.* 2004;351:1306–1313].

worsening of symptoms) may occur as the medication wears off.

Corticosteroids

Corticosteroids have become the mainstay of treatment of croup for moderate and severe disease, and even for mild disease. Steroids decrease inflammation and have been shown to decrease symptoms, decrease ED length of stay, result in decreased requirement for epinephrine, and fewer return visits to the ED. The effect is usually seen within 2 to 6 hours after administration and therefore should be given early. Intramuscular (IM), oral, and inhaled corticosteroids have all been shown to be effective in croup, with no difference in clinical efficacy between routes of administration.

Dexamethasone, as a single dose, is used most frequently because of its long half-life (approximately 54 hours). The traditional dose is 0.6 mg/kg either IM or orally. The parental formulation of dexamethasone may be given orally as it is less volume and better tolerated than the oral formulation. There is increasing evidence that lower doses may be just as effective. Other oral steroids (e.g., prednisone or prednisolone) may be given but are not as well studied and require redosing daily for 3 to 5 days because of their shorter half-life. Nebulized budesonide 2 mg has been shown to be as efficacious as oral dexamethasone

in the treatment of croup. However, since it is more expensive and less convenient to administer, it is rarely used.

Think Dehydration

Fluid requirements may be increased in children due to losses from tachypnea and fever. All children should be assessed for dehydration and their ability to tolerate oral fluids. IV fluids may be necessary.

Are Other Studies Even Necessary?

No routine laboratory tests are indicated in croup. CBC and blood culture may be indicated if there is concern for bacterial tracheitis (see Box 13-2). X-rays may reveal the classic steeple sign on the anterior-posterior (AP) view, which reflects subglottic edema (see Figure 13-1). In most cases, radiography is not indicated unless the diagnosis is in question.

Disposition

Patients should be monitored for response to therapy. The majority of patients can be discharged home from the ED. Patients with continued respiratory distress requiring multiple epinephrine nebulizers, supplemental oxygen needs, and dehydration or toxic appearance should be admitted for further treatment and evaluation.

BOX 13-2 Bacterial tracheitis

Bacterial tracheitis can mimic the symptoms of croup and is characterized by an inflammatory process of the larynx and trachea with an adherent mucopurulent membrane. Patients may have croup-like symptoms initially and then decompensate with high fever, toxic appearance, and upper airway obstruction as the membrane detaches and obstructs the airway. Children may often require intubation in order to maintain airway patency. Typical causes include *Staphylococcus aureus*, group A streptococcus, *Haemophilus influenzae* type b, *Moraxella catarrhalis*, and anaerobes. Culture of secretions should be obtained to reveal the causative agent. Treatment is with broad-spectrum antibiotics, such as oxacillin or vancomycin with ceftriaxone, in addition to anaerobic coverage if suspected.

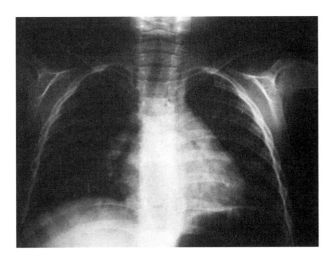

FIGURE 13-1   Croup. Steeple sign on a soft-tissue neck radiograph. (From Harwood-Nuss A, Wolfson AB, et al. *The Clinical Practice of Emergency Medicine*. 3rd ed. Philadelphia: Lippincott Williams & Wilkins; 2001.)

KEY POINTS

- Croup is an infection of the larynx, trachea, and bronchi
  - Barking cough
  - Inspiratory stridor
  - Hoarseness
  - Fever
  - Accessory muscle use
- Croup is caused by a virus
  - Parainfluenza is the most common
  - Outbreaks occur most commonly in the fall of odd-numbered years
- Subglottic edema is the cause of upper airway obstruction
  - X-ray shows the "steeple sign"
  - However, x-ray is not necessary to make the diagnosis
- Agitation and crying increase respiratory distress due to fixed upper airway obstruction
  - Minimize procedures and any other stimulation
- Treatment goal is to decrease tracheal secretions and swelling
  - Humidified oxygen increases secretion clearance
  - Epinephrine nebulizers cause vasoconstriction and resorption of edema
  - If intubation is required, anticipate difficulty due to airway narrowing
    - Endotracheal tube 0.5 to 1 mm smaller than usual should be used
- Steroids are the mainstay of treatment
  - Proven to decrease duration of symptoms
  - Dexamethasone 0.6 mg/kg given as one-time dose
    - No difference between oral and IM administration
- Most patients can be discharged home from the ED after treatment and observation
  - Observe for at least 2 hours after giving an epinephrine nebulizer
  - Rebound phenomenon is possible, although uncommon if steroids are administered

Epiglottitis

CHAPTER 14

Epiglottitis

CASE SCENARIO

A 4-year-old boy presents to the emergency department (ED) for fever and drooling. His mother states that he may have had a little runny nose yesterday but had otherwise been well. Today he had a fever to 102.4°F for which she gave Tylenol (acetaminophen). He has been very irritable and complaining of a sore throat. He also refuses to eat and has been drooling. He has no significant past medical history, takes no medication, and has no allergies. His 2-year-old sister has not been sick, nor has he had other sick contacts. He has not been fully immunized because his mother does not believe in vaccinations.

His vitals reveal a temperature of 101.6°F, pulse of 116, respiratory rate of 22, and oxygen saturation of 97%. On physical examination, he is sitting forward with his hands on his knees and his neck thrust forward and hyperextended. He looks uncomfortable but has no visible increased work of breathing.

1. What is the next step in this child's management?
   a. Examination of oropharynx
   b. Blow-by oxygen
   c. Complete blood count (CBC) and blood culture
   d. Lateral neck x-ray

This child's symptoms are concerning for epiglottitis, which is characterized by abrupt onset of fever, sore throat, dysphagia, and drooling. Children often appear toxic and they are uncharacteristically quiet and anxious-appearing. Patients are often sitting in the "tripod position," leaning forward, neck hyperextended and chin out. This position maximizes airway patency. Speech may be muffled and is referred to as "hot potato" voice as it sounds like the child is speaking with a hot object in his mouth. Respiratory distress and stridor may not be prominent.

The number-one priority is airway management. Examination of the oropharynx should not be done as it may precipitate gagging and airway closure. A lateral neck film should only be obtained if the patient is stable and the diagnosis is in question. Blood tests are not necessary to make the diagnosis. Oxygen should be given for patient comfort until appropriate actions are undertaken.

2. What is the next step in this child's management?
   a. Obtain intravenous (IV) access and start antibiotics
   b. Perform cricothyrotomy
   c. Perform endotracheal intubation
   d. Consult anesthesia for endotracheal intubation in the operating room (OR)

The most important step in the management of epiglottitis is to secure a definitive airway (i.e., endotracheal tube [ETT]), because further swelling or spasm can lead to sudden airway closure and death. This procedure should be performed in the OR by an anesthesiologist, optimally one with extensive pediatric experience, and a surgeon (either pediatric surgeon or otolaryngologist) standing by in case orotracheal intubation is impossible and a tracheostomy needs to be performed. Agitation should be minimized; therefore, IV access and antibiotics are delayed until after securing the airway. After intubation, the epiglottis can be swabbed and cultured in order to isolate a specific organism.

The patient is walked to the OR in his mother's arms. He is induced with inhaled halothane. The patient quickly falls asleep and is intubated with a 4.5 mm ETT. The anesthesiologist notes an edematous, beefy red epiglottis. Cultures are obtained and sent to microbiology. An IV is placed while the child is still under general anesthesia.

3. What is the most appropriate antibiotic regimen in this case?
   a. Ampicillin and gentamicin
   b. Vancomycin
   c. Oxacillin and ceftriaxone
   d. Levofloxacin

The antibiotic choice needs to cover the most common pathogens in epiglottitis. *Haemophilus influenzae* type b was the most common cause in the prevaccine era and still can cause disease in immunized children. It is very responsive to third-generation cephalosporins. Today, gram-positive organisms are a frequent cause, namely staphylococcus or streptococcus species. Second-generation penicillins, such as oxacillin or nafcillin, are indicated for gram-positive organisms. Therefore, the patient is given oxacillin and ceftriaxone and transferred to the pediatric intensive care unit. After 4 days of therapy, epiglottic swelling is significantly decreased and the patient is extubated. The culture grows *H. influenzae* type b sensitive to cephalosporins. The parents and his sister are given a prescription for rifampin and the child is sent home on an oral course of cefuroxime.

Answers: 1-b, 2-d, 3-c

DEFINITION

Epiglottitis refers to bacterial infection and inflammation of the epiglottis and surrounding tissues including the arytenoids, aryepiglottic folds, and the uvula. Only the supraglottic structures are affected. Edema and mucous secretion may cause aspiration or blockage of the airway, leading to respiratory arrest. Children between 1 and 5 years are most commonly affected. Typically, there is abrupt onset and rapid progression of symptoms. Epiglottitis is therefore a medical emergency and immediate evaluation and treatment is required.

ETIOLOGY

The most common cause of epiglottitis is *H. influenzae* type b (Hib). Universal immunization against Hib has had a significant impact on the incidence of disease. Other bacteria may occasionally cause epiglottitis. These include *Streptococcus pneumoniae*, group A, B or C streptococci, *Staphylococcus aureus*, *Moraxella*, *Pseudomonas*, nontypeable H. flu, and *Candida*. *Pseudomonas* and *Candida* should be suspected in immunocompromised patients. Rarely, viruses may cause epiglottitis. It has also been caused after swallowing hot tea.

MANAGEMENT

Airway—Just Leave It Alone!

The priority in management is securing the airway. Supplemental oxygen can be administered by blow-by.

LITERATURE REFERENCE

The power of immunization— No more Hib.

Epiglottitis was a common pediatric disease, mostly caused by *H. influenzae*, prior to the initiation of a vaccine against Hib. With routine universal infant immunization in the Uinted States beginning in 1991, the incidence of disease caused by *H. influenzae* type b has had a significant decrease. Infants are immunized with Hib conjugate vaccine at 2, 4, 6, and 12 to 15 months. The incidence of disease has decreased from an estimated 100 per 100,000 in the prevaccine era to 0.3 per 100,000 in 2000. Since Hib is now a rare cause of disease, epiglottitis is now uncommon [*Morb Mortal Wkly Rep.* 2002;51(11):234–237].

Agitation should be avoided as it may precipitate respiratory arrest. Emergent airway preparation should occur simultaneously. Imaging and laboratory tests should all take place after the airway is secured. In the past, most centers had an epiglottis airway team consisting of an anesthesiologist and otolaryngologist or pediatric surgeon. As it is now much less common, it may take more preparation to access these individuals. The most senior pediatrician, an anesthesiologist, and a pediatric otolaryngologist or surgeon should be called prior to intubation. Intubation should be performed in the OR under general anesthesia, where preparations can be made for a tracheostomy if intubation is unsuccessful. A tube 0.5 to 1 mm smaller than predicted (age + 16)/4 generally is used to prevent complications. After intubation, cultures of the epiglottis should be obtained by direct laryngoscopy.

Antibiotics

After the airway is secure, antibiotics should be administered. Empiric coverage should be given to cover most likely pathogens. Ceftriaxone 100 mg/kg given once a day has good gram-negative and fair gram-positive coverage and is ideal for coverage against Hib. As gram-positive organisms may be the offending agent, oxacillin or nafcillin (200 mg/kg/day in four divided doses) should be given. Given the increasing incidence of community-acquired methicillin-resistant *Staphylococcus aureus* (MRSA), the addition of vancomycin or clindamycin should be considered. Immunocompromised individuals should have therapy tailored for yeast and *Pseudomonas* infection, usually ceftazidime and fluconazole.

Imaging

X-rays should not be obtained until intubation is achieved. In young children with a hoarse voice but no other signs of epiglottitis, a portable lateral neck x-ray can be obtained. Classically, this will reveal swelling of the epiglottis (Figure 14-1), referred to as the "thumbprint sign."

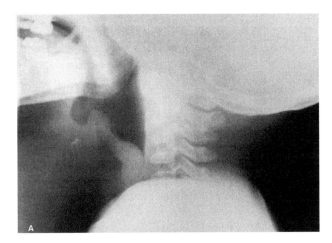

FIGURE 14-1   Epiglottitis on inspiratory soft-tissue lateral neck radiograph. (From Harwood-Nuss A, Wolfson AB, et al. *The Clinical Practice of Emergency Medicine*, 3rd ed. Philadelphia: Lippincott Williams & Wilkins; 2001)

> **BOX 14-1   Antibiotic prophylaxis for epiglottitis?**
>
> Families are often given prophylaxis if bacterial meningitis is suspected in a patient. What about epiglottitis? Invasive disease caused by *H. influenzae* type b may require prophylaxis. The American Academy of Pediatrics recommends prophylaxis for household contacts if there is one or more child less than 4 years of age who is incompletely immunized, a child younger than 12 months who has not received the primary series of immunizations, or if there is an immunocompromised child in the household. Rifampin 20 mg/kg once daily for 4 days should be prescribed.

Disposition

After securing the airway and the delivery of antibiotics, patients should be admitted to the intensive care unit (ICU) for further monitoring. Edema of the epiglottis can be monitored by direct visualization via laryngoscopy. Contacts to children with epiglottitis caused by Hib should be treated prophylactically with rifampin 20 mg/kg for 4 days (see Box 14-1).

KEY POINTS

- Epiglottitis is a true emergency as it may rapidly lead to airway closure and death
  - Avoid supine position, stimulation, or attempts at IV access
- Diagnosis is clinical
  - Toxic appearance, "tripod position", drooling, hoarse voice
  - Portable x-ray if diagnosis in doubt
    - Look for "thumbprint sign," swelling of epiglottis
- Supply blow-by supplemental oxygen
- Call most experienced clinicians for airway management
  - Intubation should occur in OR in case tracheostomy needs to be done
  - Consult anesthesiologist, and an otolaryngologist or pediatric surgeon
- *Haemophilus influenzae* type b is the most common cause of epiglottitis
  - Immunization has had a drastic effect on incidence
  - Gram-positive infection is now more common, yet still rare
    - Particularly staphylococcus and streptococcus species

- Antibiotics against gram-negative and gram-positive organisms
  - Ceftriaxone 100 mg/kg once a day PLUS
  - Oxacillin or nafcillin 200 mg/kg divided four times a day
  - Consider vancomycin or clindamycin for MRSA
- Disposition to ICU for epiglottitis or suspected epiglottitis

CHAPTER 15

Asthma

CASE SCENARIO

A 7-year-old girl is brought to the ED by ambulance for difficulty breathing. She has a history of asthma for which she has a home nebulizer machine and albuterol. She began with a runny nose 2 days ago and progressed to cough yesterday. Her mother began giving her treatments last night every 3 hours because she continued to cough and was unable to sleep. This morning her mother gave her three treatments in 1 hour because of continued cough and difficulty breathing. Her history is significant for asthma diagnosed at 4 years of age after recurrent episodes of wheezing. She has never been hospitalized and has been on steroids three times in the past, the last over a year ago. She also has a history of seasonal allergies for which she takes loratadine in the spring. She has albuterol and loratadine at home and takes no other asthma medications. She has no drug allergies. Her mother had asthma as a child that she "outgrew." There are no pets at home and they have wood floors instead of carpets. Mom occasionally smokes, but only outside. She is an only child and attends first grade.

1. What is the most concerning aspect from her initial history that suggests a more severe exacerbation?
   a. History of previous asthma attacks
   b. Prior history of steroid use
   c. Smoker in household
   d. Frequent albuterol treatments

The history is an important gauge for potential severity of disease. It is important to quantify how much and how often treatments have been given. This patient has been using multiple nebulizer treatments that are increasing in frequency, suggesting a severe exacerbation. Other pertinent history points that suggest severe disease are previous hospitalizations, ICU admissions, or intubation. Additionally, multiple recent steroid courses or noncompliance with outpatient controller medications can also predict severe disease. This is her first severe attack, she has never required hospital admission and she has infrequently required steroids. Identifying triggers for asthma exacerbations is also important. Tobacco smoke is a common trigger for worsening symptoms in asthmatics. However, while it may be a trigger in this case, in itself it does not suggest a severe exacerbation.

On physical examination, she is alert with increased work of breathing. She is unable to say more than a few words at a time and has suprasternal and intercostal retractions. Vital signs reveal a weight of 21 kg, temperature 37.6°C, heart rate (HR) 130, respiratory rate 40, and pulse oximetry of 90% on room air. On auscultation, air entry is diminished at the bases bilaterally. She has marked wheezing throughout exhalation.

2. Her skin is warm and well perfused. What is the most important next step in management?
   a. Albuterol and ipratropium nebulizer treatment
   b. Subcutaneous (SQ) epinephrine
   c. Oxygen by face mask
   d. Intravenous (IV) access and normal saline bolus

The first priority in ED management is assessment of airway, breathing, and circulation (ABCs). The patient has an intact airway (i.e., airway patent, no upper airway obstruction) but is in marked respiratory distress (i.e., lower airway obstruction, impaired ventilation). The most appropriate action is the provision of supplemental oxygen as patients with asthma develop hypoxia secondary to V/Q mismatch. Rescue therapy with a beta-agonist, albuterol, is clearly indicated in this situation but oxygen should be administered as treatment is being prepared. SQ epinephrine is an older therapy for asthma that is a nonselective beta-agonist. It has largely been replaced by SQ terbutaline, a selective β_2 agoinst. However, this is used only in severe asthma with siginificant respiratory distress. Patients with asthma exacerbations often are dehydrated secondary to tachypnea alone and may require IV fluids. Evaluation of her circulation shows good capillary refill and she does not appear cyanotic; circulation can be reassessed after managing her breathing.

Oxygen is provided by 2 liters per minute (LPM) nasal cannula and oxygen saturation improves to 94%. The patient is given an albuterol and ipratropium nebulizer treatment. Thirty minutes later, she takes off her nasal cannula and her oxygen saturation by pulse oximetry reads 88% with a HR of 138 and good waveform.

3. What is the likely cause of her worsening hypoxemia from baseline after treatment with the bronchodilator?
   a. Pneumothorax
   b. Acute respiratory distress syndrome (ARDS)
   c. Ventilation perfusion (V/Q) mismatch
   d. Pulse oximetry probe malfunction

The development of transient worsening hypoxemia may be seen after beta-agonist administration. This is caused by the inability of the medication to transit to affected airways secondary to mucus plugging and edema. Some of the medication is absorbed into the circulation and activates beta-receptors in the pulmonary arteries, increasing pulmonary blood flow to underventilated areas. Additionally, ventilated airways dilate and inflate. The result is transient worsening V/Q mismatch. Pneumothorax is a common cause of hypoxia, and can happen in asthmatics secondary to air trapping. It is not common after nebulization treatment and is more likely in asthmatics who require mechanical ventilation (i.e., positive pressure required to overcome airway obstruction can result in alveolar rupture). ARDS is seen in sepsis as a result of endotoxin-mediated destruction of the alveolar-capillary membrane. The result is diffuse alveolar exudates and progressive respiratory failure. Improper placement of the pulse oximetry probe should always be considered, especially if the distal extremities are poorly perfused and HR cannot be detected by the sensor. In this scenario, the good waveform on the monitor shows the pulse oximeter is likely correct.

The patient is placed back on supplemental oxygen by nasal cannula and is given two additional combined treatments of albuterol and ipratropium. Her breathing improves and she can now talk in full sentences. Her lung examination reveals improved aeration at the bases but continued mild expiratory wheezing. Oxygen saturation is 94% on room air. Respiratory rate has decreased to 36 per minute.

4. What further therapy is indicated in this child?
   a. Continuous albuterol therapy
   b. Oral prednisolone
   c. IV methylprednisolone
   d. IV terbutaline
   e. IV magnesium

The patient has improved significantly but still has residual mild respiratory distress. More important than the oxygen saturation is the fact that she is no longer working to breathe and can speak comfortably in complete sentences. She has tolerated time between albuterol nebulization and likely will not benefit further from continuous treatments at this time. IV terbutaline and magnesium would both be indicated if she continued to have labored breathing after serial nebulizer treatments. Steroids, such as prednisolone or methylprednisolone, are an important aspect of asthma management as they decrease inflammation; their effect is seen 4 to 6 hours after administration and they help prevent recurrence of symptoms. Both oral and IV routes have equal efficacy; therefore, the oral route is preferred. Keep in mind that children in respiratory distress have a tendency to vomit, which predisposes to aspiration. Therefore, children in moderate to severe distress should receive steroids IV.

The patient is given 40 mg of prednisolone orally and an additional albuterol treatment. She feels better but continues to have subcostal and intercostal retractions, a respiratory rate of 34, and oxygen saturation of 91% to 92% on room air. She is drinking juice, and is fully alert and interactive with her mother.

5.   What is the appropriate disposition for this child?
   a.   Admission to ICU for intensive therapy
   b.   Discharge home with home nebulizer machine
   c.   Admission to pediatric ward
   d.   Continued albuterol treatment and ED observation for the next 6 hours

The patient continues to have an oxygen requirement and requires frequent nebulizer therapy. However, it does not appear respiratory failure is imminent and she has improved. Admission to the ICU would therefore not be appropriate. Discharge home given her need for oxygen would be inappropriate, although this can be considered in asthmatics who have substantially improved after treatment in the ED. This patient should be admitted due to her persistent oxygen requirement and need for frequent nebulizers. She is discharged the next day after receiving albuterol treatments every 4 hours and receiving supplemental oxygen. She is sent home with a 5-day course of prednisone.

Answers: 1-d, 2-c, 3-c, 4-b, 5-c

DEFINITION

Asthma is a chronic obstructive lung disease characterized by episodes of reversible bronchospasm (i.e., acute airway narrowing in response to a trigger) and airway inflammation (i.e., migration of inflammatory cells with production of tissue edema and airway secretions). An asthma attack is a combination of these two processes, resulting in lower airway obstruction and manifesting as cough, wheezing, and dyspnea. Reactive airways disease (RAD) is a term often used in infants with asthma-like symptoms who do not yet have the diagnosis of asthma. Of note, bronchiolitis presents with symptoms very similar to asthma and they may be difficult to differentiate clinically as they both involve bronchiolar inflammation.

BOX 15-1   Differential diagnosis of wheezing: ABCs

- Asthma
- Anaphylaxis
- Aspiration
- Bronchiolitis
- Bronchopulmonary dysplasia (BPD)
- Cystic fibrosis
- Congenital anomalies (laryngobronchomalacia)
- Cardiac abnormalities (pulmonary edema)
- Cilia abnormalities
- Defective host (immune deficiency)
- Enlarged nodes
- Foreign body
- Gastroesophageal reflux disease (GERD)
- Infection

BOX 15-2   Risk factors for severe asthmatic disease

- Prior ICU admission
- History of intubation
- History of multiple steroid courses
- Frequent β_2-agonist use
- Rapid onset of symptoms
- Poor compliance with therapy
- Frequent emergency room visits

However, treatment for bronchiolitis is supportive and active interventions are immediately available for asthma. Asthma is the most common chronic childhood disease, with over 5 million children affected. African-Americans, those living in urban areas, and the poor are more severely affected. Boys are also more affected than girls. It is also important to remember that not all that wheezes is asthma (see Box 15-1 and Box 15-2).

ETIOLOGY

There are both genetic and environmental roles in the development of asthma. Genetics is suggested by a history of atopy (e.g., eczema, asthma, and seasonal allergies) in the patient or a family member. This can be further confirmed by laboratory testing which may reveal elevated immunoglobulin E (IgE) levels, peripheral eosinophilia, and positive skin testing. Besides genetics, multiple exposures have been implicated in asthma exacerbations. Primary allergens include dust mites, cockroach allergen, cat and

---

BOX 15-3 Deciphering the nomenclature. My baby is wheezing: Is it asthma?

There can be much confusion in the description of young children and their respiratory symptoms. Viral infections are common in young infants and more then 30% of these infections are associated with wheeze. Many of these children will have recurrent episodes of wheezing with subsequent viral illnesses; others will not. These recurrent episodes of wheezing may also last a few years and subsequently disappear as they get older. Terms such as "reactive airways disease" (RAD) and "viral-induced wheezing" are used to describe these infants in an attempt to differentiate them from true asthmatics. An episode of wheezing in an infant does not make the diagnosis of asthma. In general, infants with three or more episodes of wheezing are considered probable asthmatics. Children with recurrent wheezing from viral infections should be evaluated for other risk factors, such as history of allergies or eczema or strong family history of asthma to assess their risk of developing asthma.

---

dog allergens, fungi, and environmental tobacco smoke. Weather, exercise, psychological stress, and gastroesophageal reflux are also known triggers. Viral illnesses are the most common triggers of pulmonary symptoms in patients with known asthma. Respiratory syncytial virus (RSV) is common in young infants and rhinovirus in patients older than 3 years of age. Distinguishing viral infection from true asthma clinically can be difficult (see Box 15-3).

MANAGEMENT

Evaluation begins with assessment of ABCs. Important historical factors are duration of symptoms and possible triggers, as well as frequency of medication use since symptoms began. Respiratory distress is a term frequently used but ill-defined. It really refers to the degree a child is laboring to breathe. Signs of labored breathing, or respiratory distress, are assessed by accessory muscle use and retractions, inability to speak in full sentences, and tachypnea. Pulse oximetry is used as a measure of how well oxygen is being delivered to peripheral tissues; however, an oxygen saturation greater than 90% should not be reassuring if the child is visibly working hard to breathe. Children are notoriously able to maintain an "adequate" oxygen saturation right up to the point of sudden respiratory failure, apnea, and death. The use of peak flow meters is useful in older children and adolescents to quantify severity of airway obstruction. Dehydration is also common and fluid status should be quickly assessed.

OXYGEN AND PULSE OXIMETRY

All patients should be placed on cardiovascular monitoring and provided supplemental oxygen if evidence of respiratory distress or hypoxemia. V/Q mismatch is prominent in asthmatics and a primary cause of hypoxia. Mismatch can worsen after bronchodilator therapy as beta-agonists cause diffuse pulmonary artery dilation. This results in increased perfusion indiscriminately both to areas of adequate and inadequate ventilation, which results in V/Q mismatch.

Intubation and Ventilation

Intubation and mechanical ventilation should be avoided in asthmatics if at all possible. Therapy should concentrate on aggressive medical rescue therapy and preventing progressive respiratory failure. Indications for intubation include respiratory exhaustion leading to respiratory failure and apnea. Noninvasive mechanical ventilation may be tried initially in patients failing aggressive medical therapy through nasal continuous positive airway pressure (CPAP). If intubation is necessary, ketamine is the induction agent of choice as it has a bronchodilatory effect, although keep in mind it has been associated with laryngospasm. This however should not be an issue with the coadministration of a paralytic agent such as succinylcholine.

Cuffed endotracheal tubes should also be used to prevent air leaks around the tube as high pressures are often required for ventilation. Worsening hypoxia or increased inspiratory pressures should alert a possible complication of positive pressure ventilation, such as a pneumothorax or pneumomediastinum. Both of these conditions can quickly lead to increased intrathoracic pressures with resulting cardiac tamponade and death. A pneumothorax in this setting should be treated with needle decompression with a 16-gauge angiocatheter between the first and second ribs anteriorly, followed by placement of a chest tube.

Bronchodilators

Bronchodilators are the primary rescue therapy for asthma. The provision of a β_2-agonist results in airway smooth muscle relaxation and bronchodilatation. Beta-agonists can be delivered via intermittent or continuous nebulization, through a metered-dose inhaler (MDI) with or without a spacer, or IV. Inhaled delivery is the quickest and most effective therapy. Ideally, treatments are given every 20 minutes in the first hour and then spaced accordingly. Continuous inhalational therapy may be required in severe cases. IV administration is typically reserved for patients unresponsive to continuous nebulized therapy with impending respiratory failure.

Adequate drug delivery is an important aspect of asthma management and aerosol delivery is required to reach the lungs directly. Nebulized solution is commonly delivered in the hospital and similar devices are available for home use. It is often used in young patients as they cannot coordinate breathing for use of MDI. Nebulization requires a specialized machine to provide oxygen or compressed air to change the medication from a liquid to a small particle aerosolized form (<5 μm) to reach the smaller airways. This process takes time and can be difficult to administer in noncompliant patients. In ideal circumstances, only 10% of the medication reaches the patient's airways. Moving the delivery device even a short distance away from the airway can significantly alter the amount of medication delivered. Therefore, all nebulized medications should be delivered through a snug-fitting face mask to minimize this loss of medication delivery. Recent evidence suggests that the use of a spacer with mask is just as effective as nebulized treatment, even in young infants. The use of a spacer with a one-way valve eliminates the need

for exact coordination between the MDI puff and inhalation. The medicine remains aerosolized while the patient can breathe it in over the next few breaths.

Terbutaline is an effective IV β-agonist. SQ administration of epinephrine or terbutaline may also be reserved for cases in which IV access has not been attained. Beta-agonists result in increased adrenergic drive due to stimulation of β_1- and β_2-receptors; this is especially true with epinephrine, although the β_2-specific agents (e.g., albuterol, terbutaline) also have some cross-reactivity as well. The result is tachycardia and, rarely, tachyarrhythmias. Of note, β-receptor stimulation results in intracellular shunting of potassium. Therefore, continuous albuterol therapy can lead to hypokalemia, although the risk of arrhythmias is very low. Albuterol is the most common bronchodilator used in the emergency department (see Table 15-1 for doses of bronchodilators typically used).

Steroids

Steroids are essential in the management of asthma exacerbations, as asthma is a biphasic disease that starts with bronchospasm, followed by inflammatory cell migration, and subsequent edema and inflammation.

LITERATURE REFERENCE

Drug delivery via nebulizer versus spacer with mask

In a study of 64 children between 1 and 5 years of age with acute, recurrent wheezing, children were randomized to receive albuterol through a nebulizer (0.35 mg/kg/dose) or spacer device. The spacer device with a mask was held for eight breaths after a 50 μg/kg dose of albuterol was administered through an MDI. There was no difference in clinical efficacy as measured by the pulmonary index. In 94% of cases, parents considered administration through the spacer device easier [**Ploin D et al.** *Pediatrics.* 2000;106:311–317]. Similar efficacy was achieved in another study looking at children 2 to 24 months of age, with a suggestion of decreased hospitalization in those given medication through albuterol with spacer device [**Delgado A.** *Arch Pediatr Adolesc Med.* 2003;157:76–80]. Given its shorter administration time and ease of use, spacer and mask administration of medicine should be considered in young children in place of the nebulizer.

TABLE 15-1   Typical dosing of acute asthma medications

Drug	Formulation	Dose and route
Albuterol	0.5% (5 mg/mL) solution	0.15 mg/kg (max 5 mg) (max 5 mg) via neb q20min
	90 μg/puff MDI	1 to 2 puffs q20min
Terbutaline	1 mg/mL injectable	IV load 10 μg/kg, then continuous 0.1 μg/kg/min (max 4 μg/kg/min)
		SQ 0.01 mL/kg (max 0.3 mL)
Epinephrine	1:1,000 injectable	SQ 0.01 mL/kg (max 0.3 mL) q20min × three doses
Ipratropium bromide	250 μg/1.25 mL solution	250 μg <12 y, 500 μg >12 y via neb
	18 μg/puff aerosol	1 to 2 puffs[a]
Magnesium sulfate	Multiple	IV 25 to 75 mg/kg (max 2 g) over 20 min
Aminophylline	25 mg/mL	IV load 6 mg/kg, then continuous 1 mg/kg/h[b]

[a]Do not use aerosol ipratropium in peanut or soy allergy.
[b]Monitor levels for toxicity, goal 5 to 15 μg/mL neb, nebulizer.

Steroids decrease this second, inflammatory phase of asthma. Additionally, steroids also upregulate β_2-adrenergic receptors in bronchial smooth muscle, enhancing response to bronchodilators. Early administration of steroids is associated with decreased hospitalization, decreased length of stay, and faster resolution of symptoms. Steroids may be given orally, IV, or intramuscularly. There is no additional benefit to IV therapy and oral route is preferred in those that can tolerate it.

Various steroids can be used, the most common being oral prednisone or prednisolone and IV methylprednisolone. Doses are debated but traditionally 1 to 2 mg/kg/day. Inhaled steroids have no role in an acute asthma exacerbation but are essential in the chronic management of asthma. Short-term steroids are typically not associated with side effects. Hypertension, hyperglycemia, and mood changes may be seen, however, even with short-term use.

Anticholinergics

Anticholinergics work as bronchodilators and also decrease airway secretions. They have little value when used alone but are useful as an adjunctive

---

LITERATURE REFERENCE

Steroid dosing

Traditional dosing of oral steroids in asthma exacerbation is 1 to 2 mg/kg once or divided twice a day for 3 to 10 days. However, there may be an increase in behavioral side effects with higher doses in children. Kayani et al. performed a prospective, randomized, double-blinded study on the use of 1 mg/kg versus 2 mg/kg of oral steroids in an acute asthma exacerbation. None of the patients required hospitalization after three doses of albuterol every 20 minutes. Side effects were assessed by parent questionnaire. There was a statistically significant increased rate of anxiety and aggressive behavior in patients receiving 2 mg/kg dosing. The authors conclude that because there is no evidence of clinical difference between the two doses but there are higher rates of side effects, 1 mg/kg dosing should be used in mild asthma exacerbations [Kayani S, Shannon DC. *Chest.* 2002;122:624–628].

LITERATURE REFERENCE

Combo therapy: Ipratropium and albuterol

Considerable debate exists on the use of ipratropium in asthma exacerbations. It appears that there is significant benefit with its use in the ED. Data on the use of hospitalized patients is less clear. In one ED study, patients were randomized to receive ipratropium bromide 250 μg nebulization or normal saline (NS) with each of the first three nebulized albuterol doses. Patients receiving ipratropium resulted in the reduction in additional albuterol doses and reduced duration of treatment. There was also a lower hospitalization rate, although this was not statistically significant [Zorc JJ et al. *Pediatrics.* 1999;103:748–752]. In a meta-analysis involving the ED use of anticholinergics in asthma treatment, a subgroup analysis of pediatric studies revealed hospital admissions were reduced by 30% in the subjects that were treated with multiple doses of anticholinergic agents in addition to β_2-agonists [Bollinger MB. *Pediatrics.* 2003;112:485–486]. Qureshi et al. randomized 434 children between 2 and 18 years of age to ipratropium or NS during the second and third nebulized doses of albuterol in the ED. All patients received steroids. The rate of hospitalization was lower in the ipratropium group (27% vs. 36% in the control group). The effect was even more significant in patients with severe asthma, 37% versus 52%, respectively. [Qureshi F et al. *N Engl J Med.* 1998;339: 1030–1035]. Craven et al. looked at hospitalized children with asthma and randomized them to receive ipratropium or NS in additional to β_2-agonist therapy. There was no significant difference in length of stay or need for further therapy [Craven D et al. *Pediatrics.* 2001;138: 51–58]. Thus, ipratropium has a significant role in ED management of asthma and should be considered in all patients with moderate and severe exacerbations. Its continued use in hospitalized patients is still debatable.

treatment with β-agonists in asthma exacerbations. When combined with the administration of albuterol in the ED, significant improvement in asthmatic symptoms have been shown.

Methylxanthines

The mechanism of action of methylxanthines in asthma is unknown. They are phosphodiesterase inhibitors and thought to act as a bronchodilator and as a respiratory stimulant. Their use has become unpopular because of the narrow therapeutic range and risk of tachyarrhythmias (e.g., supraventricular tachycardia [SVT] and ventricular tachycardia [VT]) and seizures. It can also cause gastrointestinal hypermotility, with resulting abdominal pain, diarrhea, or vomiting, due to its generalized adrenergic stimulant effects. However, it may be beneficial as an adjunctive treatment in a subgroup of severe asthmatics refractory to other treatment modalities. Aminophylline can be given as an IV load 6 mg/kg, followed by continuous infusion 1 mg/kg/h to keep serum levels 5 to 15 μg/mL.

Magnesium

Magnesium, given its similar electric valence as ionized calcium, is thought to act as a competitive antagonist to calcium-mediated smooth muscle constriction. The result of "saturating" calcium receptors on smooth muscle with magnesium results theoretically in less bronchoconstriction. It has been shown effective in the treatment of moderate to severe asthma exacerbations that are refractory to serial nebulized treatments. Magnesium is given in doses 25 to 75 mg/kg (max 2 g) IV over 20 minutes every 4 to 6 hours. Toxicity includes muscle weakness, areflexia, and respiratory depression.

Fluids

Fluid management is essential, and often forgotten, in asthma. Dehydration is common due to insensible fluid losses from tachypnea as well as decreased oral intake from respiratory distress. Patients should have losses replaced and maintenance fluids provided. Oral hydration is preferred but should be avoided in those in moderate to severe distress to decrease risk of aspiration. In general, if labored breathing does not significantly improve after three albuterol nebulizers, then IV access should be obtained in case intubation or IV medications are needed. In this case, a 20 mL/kg fluid bolus should be strongly considered.

Radiography

Chest x-rays (CXR) are usually unnecessary in the management of status asthmaticus as they rarely alter therapy. Indications for CXR include first-time wheezing, a fever >39°C (102°F), lack of response to asthma therapy, or physical examination for pneumonia or other etiology of wheezing. Common CXR findings in asthma include perihilar infiltrates, hyperinflation, and atelectasis of the right middle lobe.

Peak Flow

Peak expiratory flow (PEF) is used as an objective measure of lung function in the ED and at the bedside as a substitute for formal spirometry. PEF rates correlate with spirometry measurement of forced expiratory volume. PEF is a good surrogate for the degree of airway obstruction, and it closely correlates with severity of asthma and outcome. Charts exist for predicted PEF rates for children based on height. Children 5 years or younger are usually unable to cooperate with testing. PEF is important when it can be done to follow the effectiveness of therapy.

Disposition

Many patients can be sent home from the ED with a bronchodilator and oral steroid, provided they have early follow-up with their primary care physician (PCP). Admission should be strongly considered in any patient with continued visible work of breathing (e.g., tachypnea, use of accessory muscles), oxygen saturation less than 95% on room air, or requirement of frequent nebulizer treatments (i.e., greater than every 4 hours). Patients requiring continuous nebulization therapy usually require ICU admission. Intubation should be avoided but may be necessary in patients not responding to therapy with impending respiratory failure.

KEY POINTS

- Asthma is the most common chronic disease of childhood
- Acute exacerbations present as cough, wheeze, and dyspnea
- Genetics and environment are important in disease
  - History of atopy
  - Common triggers—smoke, allergens, cockroaches, and animal dander
- Viruses are an important cause of asthma exacerbations
  - Viral-induced wheezing does not make a diagnosis of asthma
- African-Americans, the poor, and those who live in urban areas are at risk for severe disease
- History may suggest severe exacerbation
  - Onset of symptoms
  - Frequency of treatments

- Prior hospitalization, ICU, or intubation
- Poor compliance to therapy
- Physical examination focuses on evidence of labored breathing (i.e., respiratory distress)
  - Anxiety, fearful appearance
  - Use of accessory muscles
  - Tachypnea
- Provide supplemental oxygen
- Beta-agonists are first-line therapy
  - β_2-receptor stimulation results in bronchodilation
  - Albuterol (nebulized or MDI) is drug of choice
  - Terbutaline (SQ or IV) for severe disease
- Steroids are essential to decrease inflammation
  - Oral route preferred 1 mg/kg a day for mild disease
  - IV route may be necessary in severe disease due to risk of aspiration
- Anticholinergic agent ipratropium (Atrovent) used as adjunct nebulizer
  - Studies show that ED use in combination with albuterol improves symptoms
- Magnesium effective in moderate to severe disease
- Beware of dehydration and provide fluids as needed

CHAPTER 16

Bronchiolitis

CASE SCENARIO

A 3-month-old infant is brought to the ED for noisy breathing. The patient began with sneezing, runny nose, and cough 2 days ago. He has been fussy over the past day and has not been drinking much. Every time he feeds, he appears to have difficulty breathing and gets irritable. He felt warm earlier today and mom took a rectal temperature of 100.6°F. This afternoon he has had very noisy breathing and it looks like he is sucking in his belly. He is a full term infant with no previous illnesses. He attends day care 5 days a week and mom and dad smoke but only outside. There are no other children in the household and no family history of asthma, allergies, or eczema.

On examination, the infant has increased work of breathing with nasal flaring and intercostal and subcostal retractions. He appears congested with noises during inspiration and expiration. Rectal temperature is 99.6°F, heart rate is 170 beats per minute, blood pressure 80/60 mm Hg, respiratory rate 66, and pulse oximetry is 91%. Heart is regular rate and rhythm without murmur, capillary refill is < 2 seconds. He has copious nasal secretions and on auscultation of his chest you hear bilateral diffuse inspiratory crackles and rhonchi as well as expiratory wheezes. Air entry is diminished at the bases bilaterally. The patient is alert and follows you throughout the examination.

1. What is the most likely cause of this child's respiratory distress?
    a. Foreign body ingestion
    b. Upper airway obstruction
    c. Lower airway obstruction
    d. Combined upper and lower airway obstruction

The above patient presents with acute respiratory distress likely secondary to bronchiolitis. The history of illness usually begins with symptoms of rhinorrhea and cough, which usually progresses to signs of lower airway inflammation. Patients may have a low-grade fever. Bronchiolitis is caused by viral infection and spread by direct contact. Risk factors include older siblings in the house and attendance in day care. Infants that have household exposure to smoke are at risk for more severe illness. The inspiratory rhonchi reflect transmitted upper airway sounds and show some degree of upper airway obstruction. Expiratory wheezing reflects inflammation of the lower airways and obstruction of the bronchioles. While foreign body ingestion is a common cause of respiratory distress, infants typically have sudden onset of symptoms and are not otherwise ill.

2. What is the most appropriate management for this patient?
    a. Endotracheal intubation
    b. Obtain chest x-ray (CXR)
    c. Obtain vascular access and administer normal saline (NS) bolus
    d. Administer humidified oxygen

The initial management consists of assessment of airway, breathing, circulation (ABCs). Administration of supplemental oxygen is the first priority. This will help improve oxygenation, and the addition of humidified saline may help clear respiratory secretions. Use of a bulb syringe to clear nasal secretions may also be indicated in this situation. While the patient has signs of respiratory distress, he is still alert and is perfusing well. Therefore, endotracheal intubation is not indicated at this point. A CXR is not essential to establish the diagnosis and is an unnecessary delay to oxygen administration in this situation. Intravenous (IV) access is also not immediately indicated as the patient does not appear to be significantly dehydrated.

The patient is provided blow-by oxygen and has nasal secretions bulb syringed. There is some improvement in respiratory distress noted and pulse oximetry improves to 99% with supplemental oxygen.

3. What additional treatment should be administered at this point?
    a. Nebulized epinephrine
    b. Nebulized albuterol
    c. Oral prednisolone 1 mg/kg
    d. Inhaled salmeterol

Nebulized albuterol may be helpful in patients with bronchiolitis to reverse bronchospasm, especially if the child has a prior history of asthma. Similar to asthma, bronchiolitis results in lower airway obstruction, hence wheezing, as a result of airway inflammation and bronchoconstriction. Nebulized epinephrine is indicated in children with croup, but is not used in bronchiolitis. Oral steroids, such as prednisolone, have never been proven effective for children with bronchiolitis. Inhaled salmeterol is a long-acting beta-agonist that is used in older children with asthma.

Nebulized albuterol is administered; the patient is examined before and after administration. There is no improvement noted in oxygenation and the lung examination still reveals bilateral wheezes. The patient drinks 4 ounces of formula and is noted to have a wet diaper. After 4 hours of observation and several albuterol nebulizers, the patient continues to be alert and interactive, yet has moderate intercostal and subcostal retractions with a respiratory rate in the 60s and an oxygen saturation of 90% to 93% on room air.

4. What is the appropriate disposition for this patient?
    a. Admit to general pediatric floor for supplemental oxygen
    b. Admit to pediatric ICU for closer monitoring
    c. Discharge home with home nebulizer machine and albuterol nebulizers
    d. Discharge home with primary care follow-up the next day

This patient continues to have moderate respiratory distress with decreased oxygen saturations. He is otherwise alert and drinking well. This patient requires admission for further observation, supplemental oxygen, and further breathing treatments. While the patient may continue to deteriorate, he currently is not in severe enough distress to warrant ICU admission. Young children are at risk for respiratory failure and apnea so they should be observed in the hospital if they are working to breathe or have impaired oxygenation.

Answers: 1-d, 2-d, 3-b, 4-a

DEFINITION

Bronchiolitis refers to a lower respiratory tract infection with inflammation of the bronchioles. Bronchiolar inflammation leads to increased edema and mucus plugging, causing airway narrowing. Clinically, patients usually begin with rhinorrhea and cough and progress to tachypnea, increased work of breathing, and wheezing. Typically, it affects young children with small airways; therefore, children under 2 years of age are commonly affected. Younger children may have more severe disease, and newborns may present with apnea. Mortality is highest in premature infants, those with congenital heart disease or immune deficiency, and those less than

BOX 16-1   Indications for hospitalization in bronchiolitis
● Age <3 months
● Prematurity
● Congenital heart disease
● Saturation <95% by pulse oximetry
● Respiratory rate >70
● Atelectasis on CXR
● Ill or toxic appearing
● Inadequate fluid intake

6 weeks of age. Bronchiolitis is the most common cause of hospitalization in infants (see Box 16-1).

ETIOLOGY

Bronchiolitis is caused by a viral infection, most commonly respiratory syncytial virus (RSV). RSV is spread primarily through contact with nasal secretions. The remainder of cases is caused by other viruses, including parainfluenza, adenovirus, influenza, and rhinovirus. A new virus, human metapneumovirus, has recently been described as a cause of RSV-negative bronchiolitis. *Chlamydia trachomatis* and *Mycoplasma pneumoniae* may cause similar illnesses. Seasonal variation in bronchiolitis is determined by the etiologic agent; RSV causes fall and winter epidemics, parainfluenza more likely spring epidemics.

MANAGEMENT

A Clinical Diagnosis with Few Proven Therapies

The diagnosis of bronchiolitis is clinical and the management is supportive. Laboratory and radiographic studies may support the diagnosis or help in eliminating a fever workup in a young infant but are not necessary to make the diagnosis. There are multiple therapies offered for bronchiolitis, although their efficacy is controversial. Oxygen and fluids remain the mainstay of therapy. Initial and adequate assessment of ABCs is the most important step in management. Patients in severe respiratory distress or apnea may require intubation and mechanical ventilation. IV fluids should be considered for all patients with poor oral intake, given the increased insensible losses due to hyperventilation and fever.

Radiographs

CXR commonly reveals hyperinflation and peribronchial cuffing. Airway inflammation and edema may lead to mucus plugging and areas of atelectasis. These areas may be mistaken for infiltrates, and antibiotics are often unnecessarily given. Similar to asthma, a CXR is not helpful in making the diagnosis of bronchiolitis, and it is only indicated in cases of severe respiratory distress or suspected bacterial coinfection (e.g., fever, toxic appearance, and significant hypoxia). There is little correlation between CXR findings and disease severity in bronchiolitis.

Laboratory workup

Laboratory workup, including complete blood count (CBC) and blood cultures should be obtained according to the fever algorithms presented in Chapters 7 and 8. As demonstrated by Levine et al. (see LR in Chapter 7, p 44.), RSV-positive infants less than 28 days of age with a fever still require a full sepsis workup due to the incidence of serious bacterial illness (SBI) of about 10%. In the 29 to 60 day age-group, the incidence of SBI fell to about 5% in Levine's study, with many coincident urinary tract infections (UTIs), emphasizing the importance of urinalysis and culture in this age group. However, given the still-significant incidence of SBI in this age group, a full sepsis evaluation is recommended even if the infant presents clinically as bronchiolitis. Based on the fever algorithms, febrile infants between the ages of 60 days to 6 months should have a basic workup of CBC, blood culture, and urinalysis. After 6 months, fever in the setting of clinical bronchiolitis is rarely SBI. A nasal wash should be obtained in infants with suspected bronchiolitis. Rapid detection antigen tests exist for RSV, as well as for influenza, parainfluenza, and adenovirus that can confirm the diagnosis of viral bronchiolitis.

Oxygen Is Key

Pulse oximetry should be done to follow the degree of hypoxemia. Supplemental oxygen can be provided by nasal prongs, face mask, or blow-by. Humidified oxygen may be helpful or patients may

LITERATURE REFERENCE

Risk of serious bacterial illness (SBI) with RSV infection

With RSV often associated with fever, an often-asked question is whether to rule out SBI in children under 3 years of age with fever and clinical evidence of bronchiolitis. Patients under 3 months are at highest risk for sepsis and are commonly infected with RSV. In a retrospective analysis, Melendez and Harper looked at the utility of a sepsis evaluation in infants under 90 days of age. Of 329 infants with clinical bronchiolitis, there were no cases of bacteremia or meningitis. Only 2% had positive urine cultures, several of which were likely contaminants. However, only 57% received full sepsis workup in this study, so some bacterial infections may have been missed. This study suggests that infants younger than 90 days with fever and clinical bronchiolitis may not need a full sepsis workup **[Melendez E and Harper MB. *Pediatr Infect Dis J.* 2003;22:1053–1056]**.

Kupperman et al. conducted a prospective trial looking at children under 2 years of age with fever, with and without clinical signs of bronchiolitis. The rate of bacteremia was 0% in the bronchiolitis-with-fever group and 2.7% in the fever-only group. The rate of UTI was 1.9% and 13.6%, respectively **[Kupperman N et al. *Arch Pediatr Adolesc Med.* 1997;151:1207–1214]**. Purcell et al. performed a retrospective analysis of 2,396 hospitalized infants for RSV bronchiolitis and recorded the rate of bacterial infection. There were 39 positive cultures (1.6%), 12 were positive blood cultures, all of which were likely contaminants. The remaining 27 were all positive urinary tract cultures with typical pathogens. Eliminating the contaminants, the true rate of bacterial illness, all UTIs, was 1.1% **[Purcell K et al. *Arch Pediatr Adolesc Med.* 2002; 156:322–324]**. From the data it seems reasonable to obtain a urinalysis and culture in children older than 6 months with bronchiolitis and fever, and that a blood culture is unnecessary in nontoxic-appearing children. For those <6 months, a fever must be worked up more extensively, even in the face of clinical bronchiolitis.

LITERATURE REFERENCE

Bronchodilators and bronchiolitis: Lots of studies, few conclusions

There continues to be controversy regarding the effective management of bronchiolitis. Part of the controversy resides in the fact that infants with bronchiolitis present similarly to older children with viral-induced RAD with respiratory distress, wheezing, and recent viral infection. However, the pathogeneses of these two diseases are distinct and it is not surprising that the response to therapy may be different. Patel et al. looked at the effectiveness of epinephrine, albuterol, or placebo (normal saline) nebulization in infants with bronchiolitis randomized from the ED. There was no difference in length of stay, time to normal oxygenation, time to adequate oral intake, or mean time to decreased respiratory distress. However, a majority of patients had received an albuterol nebulization and one-third of patients had received an epinephrine nebulization prior to randomization, with unknown effect on outcome **[Patel H et al. *J Pediatr.* 2002;141:818–824]**. A Cochrane database meta-analysis of randomized trials using bronchodilators found 8 trials totaling 394 children. There was noted to be some improvement in clinical scores of some patients receiving albuterol; however, this may have been confounded by the addition of recurrent wheezing in some of the trials. There was no difference in rate of hospitalization, length of stay, or oxygenation requirement **[Kellner JD et al. *Cochrane Database Syst Rev.* 2005;1:CD001266]**. Despite this, bronchodilators are commonly used in the treatment of bronchiolitis, especially if the child has a history of wheezing.

be placed in mist tents to enhance mucus clearance. Rarely is intubation required in bronchiolitis.

Bronchodilators—Sometimes They Work and Sometimes They Don't

Accumulated data from randomized trials and meta-analyses do not per se support the use of bronchodilators (i.e., nebulized albuterol) in bronchiolitis, yet they are frequently used anyway. While some meta-analyses have revealed benefit, they also did not account for wheezing caused by bronchiolitis versus viral-induced asthma exacerbations. A subset of patients with episodes of recurrent wheezing may have effective relief from bronchodilators. For this reason, patients with a history of recurrent wheezing or a strong family history of atopy, such as asthma, seasonal allergies, or eczema, are often given a trial of a bronchodilator and monitored for clinical response. If improvement is noted within one hour, therapy is often continued as needed.

Epinephrine—Used Infrequently in Bronchiolitis

Epinephrine is considered in bronchiolitis because of its combined α- and β-adrenergic effects. While the β-adrenergic effects are similar to albuterol, the α-adrenergic stimulation causes vasoconstriction and may help decrease edema and subsequent mucus plugging that is prominent in bronchiolitis. Similar to albuterol, meta-analyses have demonstrated lack of clear benefit of inhaled epinephrine in bronchiolitis. While multiple studies show a beneficial effect on heart rate, respiratory rate, and oxygen requirement after 1 hour, no impact on the rate of hospitalization or length of hospital stay has been consistently documented. Nevertheless, nebulized epinephrine may be helpful for children with severe respiratory distress, and some clinicians use it routinely in this subgroup of children.

Steroids Are Useless for Bronchiolitis

Corticosteroids have anti-inflammatory effects and are thought to decrease bronchiolar swelling and thus airway obstruction. Steroids have been used in the past for bronchiolitis; however, the current consensus is that they have no utility. Many studies are again complicated by the inclusion of patients with multiple episodes of prior wheezing who may be more steroid-responsive. Meta-analysis has revealed little difference in hospitalization rate or length of stay in children with bronchiolitis given steroids. Patients with severe disease who require mechanical ventilation have also shown variable effect with some studies showing decreased days of ventilation while others show no benefit. The bottom line is that steroids are not used in bronchiolitis.

LITERATURE REFERENCE

Epinephrine and bronchiolitis: The same outcome

A randomized trial involving 194 infants using epinephrine versus placebo in bronchiolitis found that there was no significant change in respiratory rate or effort after treatment, although an increase in heart rate was noted **[Wainwright C et al. *N Engl J Med.* 2003;349:27–35]**. A meta-analysis of epinephrine again found conflicting results on benefit. Fourteen studies were found, involving both inpatients and outpatients. Among inpatients, nebulized epinephrine was only found to have improved clinical score at 60 minutes compared to placebo and improved respiratory rate at 30 minutes compared to albuterol. Among outpatients, epinephrine treatment was noted to have improved clinical score, oxygenation and respiratory rate at 30 minutes compared to placebo and improved oxygenation at 60 minutes; heart rate at 90 minutes and respiratory rate at 60 minutes compared to albuterol. However, there was no difference in rate of hospitalization among outpatients **[Hartling L et al. *Cochrane Database Syst Rev.* 2005;1:CD003123]**. The benefit of bronchodilators remains unclear at this time. There may be some benefit with albuterol in patients with recurrent wheezing, suggesting a bronchospastic component. Epinephrine may have some benefit in reducing edema and respiratory distress in bronchiolitis, although improvement has not been consistently documented. Like bronchodilators, epinephrine is used, albeit less frequently, in the treatment of bronchiolitis.

Antibiotics or Antivirals Indicated?

Antibiotics should only be administered if there is a clear source of bacterial infection or the child is toxic-appearing. Pneumonia should be suspected in infants with a high fever (temperature >39°C) and tachycardia or hypoxia; antibiotics can be administered if an infiltrate is present on CXR. In addition to bacterial pneumonia, otitis media can be a complication of viral bronchiolitis that would require antibiotics. The vast majority of cases of bronchiolitis, however, do not require antibiotics. Antiviral therapy with ribavirin, a nucleoside analogue, is available for patients with RSV bronchiolitis. However, data again is conflicting, and its high cost and difficulty in administration prohibits its use in most cases.

Most Will Be Dehydrated

Assessment of circulation and hydration status is critical. Infants may have increased insensible losses with elevated respiratory rates, and this is especially so with bronchiolitis. Additionally, fever may increase metabolic demands and fluid requirements. Patients may have difficulty taking in fluids given the degree of upper airway obstruction or respiratory distress. Oral intake and wet diapers should be assessed and documented. IV hydration should be considered in all patients if fluid intake is inadequate and signs of dehydration exist (e.g., sallow appearance, dry mucous membranes, decreased urine output [UOP]).

An Ounce of Prevention

As the treatment is supportive and few effective interventions exist, strategies to prevent RSV bronchiolitis in high-risk infants are important. Immunoprophylaxis with a humanized monoclonal antibody against RSV (palivizumab) may be given to certain infants under 2 years of age via an intramuscular (IM) injection monthly during winter months (see Box 16-2). Respiratory syncytial immune globulin intravenous (RSV-IVG) contains high titers of neutralizing RSV antibody but must be given IV and is currently not the preferred method of prophylaxis. All high-risk patients should be asked on ED visits whether they are receiving their monthly RSV prophylaxis during the winter months.

KEY POINTS

- Bronchiolitis is a viral infection causing inflammation of the bronchioles
  - Children under 2 years of age are primarily affected
  - Beware of severe course if age < 6 weeks, premature, or comorbid illness
- RSV is the most common cause of bronchiolitis
  - Influenza, parainfluenza, and adenovirus are also common causes
  - Human metapneumovirus is a new virus that also is a common cause
- Symptoms include nasal congestion, cough, and difficulty breathing
  - Fever may be present
  - Younger children are at risk for apnea
- Chest x-ray is not necessary for the diagnosis
  - Atelectasis is a common finding
- Risk of SBI in bronchiolitis is relatively low
  - Fever workup per fever algorithm for age < 6 months
  - No fever workup if > 6 months, although still consider urinalysis (UA) in girls
- Rapid antigen tests for RSV exist to confirm the diagnosis
- Treatment is supportive
  - Humidified oxygen
  - Albuterol nebulization, especially if prior history of wheezing or family history of atopy
  - Epinephrine nebulization transiently improves oxygenation
    - However, it has little effect on course of disease and is not typically used
  - Steroids are not recommended
  - Antibiotics are not indicated unless superimposed SBI or otitis media suspected
  - Antiviral therapy is expensive and has not shown proven benefit
- Prophylaxis available with palivizumab (monoclonal antibody against RSV)
  - Infants with prematurity, chronic lung disease, congenital heart disease

---

BOX 16-2   Prevention of RSV through palivizumab prophylaxis. Who should be getting it?

RSV prophylaxis with monthly intramuscular injections of immunoglobulin, palivizumab, during RSV season decreases the risk of hospitalizations in infants with chronic lung disease, prematurity, and congenital heart disease. These groups of patients are at increased risk for severe disease and death from RSV infection. Indications for prophylaxis are children < 2 years of age with chronic lung disease requiring medical therapy, infants born at < 32 weeks if RSV season within 6 months, infants born at < 28 weeks if RSV season within 12 months, and infants born at 32 to 35 weeks if they have more than two of the following risk factors: attendance at day care, school age siblings, smokers in household, congenital airway abnormalities, or neuromuscular disease. Children with hemodynamically significant cyanotic and acyanotic heart disease (i.e., requires medication for congestive heart failure, or has pulmonary hypertension) should also receive prophylaxis. It is not indicated in patients with small atrial sepal defect (ASDs) or ventricular septal defect (VSDs), mild pulmonary stenosis, patent ductus arteriosus (PDA), or mild coarctation.

CHAPTER 17

Congenital Heart Disease

CASE SCENARIO

A 1-year-old infant arrives in the ED by ambulance with a reported "blue" spell at home. Her parents do not speak English and are therefore unable to provide any further history without an interpreter. The paramedics report that when they arrived at the house, the patient was quiet and sleeping on her stomach with her knees at her chest. On arrival to the ED, her vital signs include a pulse of 140, blood pressure of 85/40, respiratory rate of 32, and arterial oxygen saturation (SaO_2) of 89%. On physical examination, she appears small for her age, but is sleeping without distress. Her cardiac examination reveals a loud 3/6 systolic murmur heard best at the left upper sternal border and a single second heart sound. Her lungs are clear and there is no hepatomegaly or digital clubbing. Her femoral pulses are palpable.

1. Which congenital cardiac lesion do you suspect?
   a. Transposition of the great arteries (TGA)
   b. Tricuspid atresia
   c. Truncus arteriosus (TA)
   d. Tetralogy of Fallot (TOF)

All of the above congenital cardiac anomalies cause cyanosis. Transposition typically presents early in the neonatal period as the ductus arteriosus closes. Truncus often presents in the first several weeks of life with signs and symptoms of heart failure due to high-pressure left ventricular blood flow into the pulmonary arteries. Tricuspid atresia also typically presents very early in life; however, if the associated ventricular septal defect (VSD) is relatively large and pulmonary blood flow is adequate, an infant may not present until the first several years of life. Similarly, TOF can also present at variable ages depending on the degree of pulmonic stenosis. In cases of severe pulmonic stenosis, patients will present early in the neonatal period as the ductus closes. If the degree of pulmonic stenosis is less severe, patients may present over the course of the first several years of life as the right ventricular outflow tract obstruction progressively worsens.

2. What ECG findings would you most likely see in this condition?
   a. Left axis deviation
   b. Left ventricular hypertrophy
   c. Right ventricular hypertrophy
   d. Right atrial enlargement

Right ventricular hypertrophy (RVH) is always seen with TOF secondary to the VSD and its predominating left to right shunt, which increases the total volume of blood seen by the right ventricle. RVH also develops secondary to variable degrees of right ventricular outflow tract obstruction. This occurs at the level of the infundibulum, or base, of the pulmonic valve. It can also extend to the level of the pulmonary artery and cause severe pulmonary artery stenosis or atresia. The obstruction is typically progressive, and therefore children who are "pink" at birth may progress to have cyanotic episodes as the obstruction worsens. Right atrial enlargement (RAE) is often, but not always, seen with TOF, most often occurring in children who present outside of the neonatal period. Right axis deviation, not left, is seen due to the increased forces in the right side of the heart.

While performing an ECG, which reveals both RVH and borderline RAE, the patient wakes and begins to cry inconsolably. She develops central cyanosis and concordantly her oxygen saturation drops to 72%. You again listen to her precordium and note that the murmur has disappeared. At this point, your suspicion for TOF is very high given her murmur, which is consistent with pulmonic stenosis and which disappears in the setting of cyanosis, the ECG findings, and the intermittent cyanotic episodes. You place the child in a knee-to-chest position over her father's shoulder and provide supplemental oxygen.

3. What is the next step in her management?
   a. Administer prostaglandin E (PGE) 0.1 mcg/kg/min
   b. Intubate
   c. Administer Lasix (furosemide) 1 mg/kg IV
   d. Administer morphine 0.1 mg/kg SQ/IM

"Tet spells" are characterized by the acute development of cyanosis during circumstances that further decrease the already compromised pulmonary blood flow in patients with TOF. Typically spells occur in the setting of increased pulmonary pressures (crying) and/or decreased peripheral vascular resistance (bathing, fever, or exercise). Under either of these circumstances, blood travels down the pressure gradient (from areas of relatively high to low pressure) and thus unsaturated blood shunts from right to left across the VSD, creating cyanosis. The treatment for such spells is to reverse the abnormal cardiac physiology by increasing pulmonary blood flow and/or increasing peripheral vascular resistance so that blood shunts from the left ventricle through the VSD into the right ventricle and on through the pulmonary vasculature to become oxygenated in the lungs.

Your first priority is to try to calm the child and minimize agitation while providing basic support. Therefore, the patient should be kept in the company of her parents and any noxious stimuli, such as blood draws or IV attempts, should be avoided initially if possible. Oxygen is a must, but should be administered in the least invasive manner possible, typically via open tubing and not via a face mask. The knee-to-chest position is helpful by increasing peripheral vascular resistance, decreasing the right-to-left shunt, and increasing pulmonary blood flow. Parenteral morphine is effective for several reasons. First, it helps calm the child and reduce her oxygen consumption and tachypnea. It also dilates the pulmonary arteries and therefore reduces resistance to the right-sided outflow tract.

Prostaglandin administration in a neonate helps prevent closure of the ductus arteriosus. Thus, it is a very useful drug to administer when a neonate presents with cyanosis and there is concern for a ductal-dependent cardiac lesion. However, by the end of the first year of life, the ductus is most likely either closed or fixed open. It would be extremely unlikely for it to close abruptly after one year without medical or surgical intervention. Thus, a closing ductus is not likely responsible for this patient's cyanosis and, therefore, prostaglandin is not indicated. Lasix is not indicated in this situation, as pulmonary edema is not the reason for increased pulmonary vascular resistance. Intubation and mechanical ventilation would cause an increase in pulmonary vascular pressure and result in an increase in the right-to-left shunt.

4. After 5 minutes, the infant remains cyanotic and restless. What is your next step?
   a. Phenylephrine IV 0.02 mg/kg
   b. 20 cc/kg NS bolus with sodium bicarbonate administration
   c. Propranolol IV 0.1 mg/kg
   d. Arrange for emergency corrective surgery

The administration of fluids with bicarbonate should be initiated to counteract the ensuing acidosis. Additional intravascular volume will also increase the systemic blood pressure and help reverse the shunting pattern during a spell. An alpha-agonist, such as phenylephrine, can be helpful as it will increase systemic vascular resistance (SVR) by causing peripheral vasoconstriction, but it is not the first-line intervention. Propranolol also plays a role in management of TOF. It is thought to decrease the degree of infundibular spasm thereby decreasing the degree of right ventricular outflow tract obstruction and favoring blood flow through the pulmonary circuit. Emergency palliative shunt surgery is rarely required, but if symptoms persist for > 30 minutes and if the previously mentioned interventions are not successful at reducing the degree of right-to-left shunting across the VSD, then surgery may be required urgently to create an artificial shunt between the systemic vasculature (typically the right subclavian artery) and the pulmonary artery to restore blood flow to the lungs and reverse the hypoxia and acidosis.

While you are placing the IV for administration of fluids and medication, you obtain a venous blood gas (VBG), electrolytes, and a complete blood count (CBC).

5. Which of the following would be inconsistent with the patient's clinical picture?
   a. Hematocrit of 55%
   b. Bicarbonate of 13
   c. Mixed venous oxygen saturation (SvO$_2$) of 80
   d. Anion gap of 24

Polycythemia (increased hematocrit) is often seen in patients with chronic hypoxia and therefore is not uncommon in patients with TOF who persistently have some degree of mixing between oxygenated and unoxygenated blood. The low bicarbonate is expected and represents a metabolic acidemia, resulting from decreased oxygen delivery to the tissues and the resulting anaerobic metabolism with release of lactic acid. The increased anion gap is also consistent with ongoing anaerobic metabolism and a build up of lactate. The mixed venous oxygen saturation (SvO$_2$) would be much lower than 80 (normal range 70 to 100 mm Hg), given the fact that it is from a venous sample and given the degree of cyanosis.

By this time, an interpreter has arrived. You are not surprised to learn that your young patient has had multiple similar episodes in her short life and her parents confirm her diagnosis of TOF. They report that she had been on medication for this condition, you suspect a β-blocker, but they had run out 2 weeks ago and had not yet refilled her prescription. They inform you that she is scheduled for corrective surgery in 3 weeks.

Answers: 1-d, 2-c, 3-d, 4-b, 5-c

True Blue—Central versus Acral Cyanosis

Cyanosis describes a bluish hue to the skin, mucous membranes, and nail beds. When cyanosis is isolated to the hands and feet, it is referred to as acrocyanosis. Acrocyanosis results from peripheral vascular constriction in newborns, which occurs as part of normal transitioning from intrauterine to extrauterine life. Acrocyanosis is extremely common in neonates and can persist for several days. When cyanosis involves the mucous membranes (e.g., buccal mucosa) and lips it is referred to as central, and is always pathologic. Central cyanosis occurs when the amount of oxygen added to circulation via ventilation is less than the amount of oxygen removed from hemoglobin for cellular activity. There are many different causes for imbalances in this equation, but this discussion will focus on cyanosis resulting from congenital cardiac lesions, which result from various embryologic errors in cardiac development (see Box 17-1).

A Quick Review of Fetal Circulation

The fetus depends on oxygenated blood from its mother via the umbilical vein, which then joins with the inferior vena cava (IVC) via the ductus venosus. The majority of oxygenated blood that enters the right atrium (RA) from the IVC is preferentially shunted across the foramen ovale into the left atrium and then on to the systemic circulation via the left ventricle and aorta. A small portion of blood, mostly deoxygenated, travels from the RA to the right ventricle and into the pulmonary artery. Because of the high pulmonary pressures in the fetus, this small volume of blood in the pulmonary artery is shunted across the ductus arteriosus into the aorta and systemic circulation.

Following birth this circulation pattern changes rather abruptly. Under normal circumstances, the foramen ovale and ductus arteriosus close within the first 24 to 48 hours of life, thus obliterating shunting between the right and left atria and pulmonary artery and aorta, respectively. This is a critical time for infants with congenital cardiac defects that depend on the ductus arteriosus for either pulmonary or systemic blood flow, and thus a common time for neonates to develop cyanosis and present emergently for evaluation and treatment (see Box 17-2).

What to Do for a Baby Who Is Blue

The initial care of any cyanotic patient begins with an evaluation of the airway, breathing, and circulation (ABCs). If the patient is breathing with a stable airway, then immediate intubation should not be performed even in the setting of severe cyanosis until a thorough physical examination, chest x-ray, and ECG have been obtained to help differentiate the reason behind the cyanosis. The top three most worrisome causes for cyanosis in a newborn include sepsis,

---

BOX 17-1 Why so blue? When what goes in does not equal what comes out

Not Enough In

- Apnea
  - Neurologic: CNS dysfunction (intracranial hemorrhage, seizures) or neuromuscular dysfunction (botulism, neonatal myasthenia gravis)
  - Pharmacologic
- Diffusion problem: surfactant deficiency (neonatal RDS), retained fetal lung fluid or transient tachypnea of the newborn (TTN), pneumonia, pulmonary hypoplasia, congenital cystic adenomatoid malformation (CCAM)
- Obstruction
  - Extrinsic: pneumothorax, chylothorax, hemothorax, vascular ring or pulmonary sling
  - Intrinsic: laryngo/tracheo/bronchomalacia, bronchiolitis, croup, pertussis

Poor oxygenation

- Shunting lesions
  - Cardiac: TOF, pulmonic atresia, tricuspid atresia, TGA with intact ventricular septum, Ebstein anomaly, truncus arteriosus, Eisenmenger syndrome
  - Non-cardiac: persistent pulmonary hypertension of the newborn (PPHN)
- Hematologic: methemoglobinemia, carboxyhemoglobinemia

Too Much Out

- High oxygen consumption
  - Sepsis!
- Low flow state—high level of oxygen extraction with decreased cardiac output
  - Hypoplastic left heart, coarctation of the aorta, TAPVR with obstruction
  - Cardiomyopathy, myocarditis, polycythemia (high viscosity)

CNS, central nervous system; RDS, respiratory distress syndrome.

BOX 17-2 Who needs a patent ductus anyway?

Lesions dependent on left-to-right shunting through ductus

- Tricuspid atresia
- Pulmonic atresia
- TOF with severe right outflow tract obstruction
- Ebstein anomaly

Lesions dependent on right-to-left shunting through ductus

- Hypoplastic left heart syndrome
- Interrupted aortic arch
- Critical coarctation of the aorta
- TAPVR with obstruction

---

congenital heart disease (CHD), and congenital adrenal hyperplasia (CAH). The distinction between these three diagnoses is not always straightforward, but the physical examination is the first place to start to look for clues to help with the differentiation.

The physical examination should start with review of the vital signs. Preductal (right hand) and postductal (left hand or feet) simultaneous pulse oximetry saturations should be obtained early in the evaluation process. If there is a discrepancy of more than 5% across the two measurements, then a cardiac etiology should be suspected. Higher preductal saturations indicate that deoxygenated blood from the pulmonary artery is shunting to the aorta. When the postductal saturation is significantly higher than the preductal, the suspicion for transposition of the great arteries (TGA) should be high. The cardiac examination is important in differentiating congenital cardiac lesions as is detailed later in the chapter (see Box 17-3). Pathologic murmurs however must be distinguished from normal, physiologic murmurs. In general, the latter tend to be soft, of short duration, and early in systole. Pathologic murmurs tend to be loud, long, and in various parts of the cardiac cycle depending on the lesion.

Supplemental oxygen therapy should be provided cautiously for cyanotic patients in whom congenital heart disease is suspected, as oxygen accelerates the closure of the ductus. Therefore, some recommend that supplemental oxygen be held until prostaglandin administration has been started. Others recommend that minimal oxygen be provided and that saturations as low as 75% should be tolerated when suspicious of cyanotic congenital heart disease (CCHD), until a definitive diagnosis can be made. Thus, if you decide to initiate oxygen therapy, and subsequently a patient has

---

BOX 17-3 Listen for your diagnosis

Many useful clues that will lead you to a more specific diagnosis within the realm of cyanotic congenital heart disease can be obtained with your stethoscope. Specifically, paying close attention to the second heart sound will help you to differentiate between lesions that result in increased or decreased flow through the pulmonary circuit. In lesions which have very little or no flow through the pulmonary artery (tricuspid or pulmonic atresia, and TOF with severe right outflow tract obstruction) only a single second heart sound will be appreciated. This represents the closing of the aortic valve in the absence of pulmonic valve closure. Lesions with increased pulmonary blood flow, are characterized by a widely split S2 which does not vary significantly with respiration. Such lesions include TAPVR, TA, TGA, ASDs, or VSDs.

worsening respiratory distress or decreased peripheral perfusion, think of ductal-dependent disease and stop oxygen and give prostaglandin emergently. Oxygen therapy is also traditionally used to help differentiate between cardiac and noncardiac etiologies for cyanosis. The hyperoxia test is one method used to differentiate between pulmonary and cardiac etiologies of cyanosis (see Box 17-4).

Echocardiography is the gold standard of diagnosis, as it is a non-invasive technique that identifies cardiac anatomy as well as additional information regarding flow patterns. If echocardiogram reveals a ductal-dependent lesion, or if the collective findings from the patient's physical examination, ECG, and chest x-ray are suspicious for cardiac anomalies, then a cardiologist should be consulted to provide guidance regarding

---

BOX 17-4   Where's the problem? Use the hyperoxia test to guide you

The hyperoxia test is useful, although not absolute, in differentiating cardiac disease from pulmonary disease. The basic premise behind the test is that no amount of supplemental oxygen will significantly increase the partial pressure of oxygen in arterial blood (PaO_2) in a shunting lesion where blood never flows through the lungs. To perform the test, first draw a baseline ABG while the infant is breathing room air. Next administer 100% oxygen for at least 10 minutes, and subsequently draw another ABG and compare results.

In the presence of pulmonary disease (e.g., TTN, pneumonia, RDS), the PaO_2 should rise by at least 30 to 100 mm Hg over the baseline value. In the presence of cardiac disease, specifically cyanotic or mixed flow defects, the rise in PaO_2 is minimal, typically < 30 mm Hg. This test should be interpreted with caution, however. Oxygen alone may be insufficient to correct hypoxemia in newborns with right-to-left shunting due to persistent pulmonary hypertension or severe ventilation-perfusion mismatching due to severe pneumonia or severe meconium aspiration syndrome. In such patients with severe pulmonary disease higher oxygen content often needs to be delivered via continuous positive airway pressure or positive-pressure ventilation.

But don't be fooled, there are also cyanotic cardiac lesions which may be missed with this test early on while the ductus arteriosus remains patent. Specifically, neonates with transposition of the great arteries and PPHN may have a PaO_2 that increases significantly with 100% supplemental oxygen. This is because the high pulmonary pressures favor the flow of oxygenated blood from the left heart circuit into the right heart circuit, which in this scenario is the systemic circulation. Patients with TAPVR or hypoplastic left heart may also have a PaO_2 more than 100 mm Hg with a patent ductus in 100% supplemental oxygen.

BOX 17-5   When should I use prostaglandin-E1?

Prostaglandin-E1 (PGE1) causes vasodilation of all arterioles and therefore can be useful in maintaining patency of the ductus arteriosus. In short, PGE1 administration in a cyanotic newborn can be lifesaving! It should be thought of very early in the evaluation of any infant who presents in the first week of life with a history and physical examination suggestive of cardiac disease. The risk-benefit ratio is low with the three most common side effects including hyperpyrexia, apnea, and flushing. The common starting dose for a PGE1 continuous infusion is 0.1 mcg/kg/min. Close CVR monitoring is essential and prophylactic intubation should be strongly considered given the possibility of apnea, particularly in a patient who requires transport between facilities.

---

prostaglandin administration in an effort to maintain patency of the ductus arteriosus (see Box 17-5).

The 5 Ts

The classic teaching for CCHD includes the 5 Ts, referring to TOF, tricuspid atresia, total anomalous pulmonary venous return (TAPVR), TA, and TGA. Pulmonic atresia is a sixth lesion which will also be included in this discussion as it, similar to TOF and tricuspid atresia, results in right-sided outflow obstruction to the pulmonary arteries and thus a right-to-left shunting of venous blood in the heart. This results in decreased pulmonary blood flow, decreased rate of oxygen transfer across alveolar capillary beds, and thus cyanosis. In contrast to the above lesions, TAPVR, TA, and TGA, as well as isolated atrial septal defects (ASDs) and VSDs, all result in increased pulmonary blood flow that predispose to congestive heart failure (see Box 17-6 and Table 17-1.)

BOX 17-6   What else can go wrong? Extracardiac manifestations of cyanotic congenital heart disease

- Polycythemia is induced by chronic hypoxia
- Brain abscesses are more common due to right-to-left shunting
- Thromboembolisms are more common due to the increased blood viscosity caused by polycythemia and they tend to travel directly to the brain in the presence of right-to-left shunting which bypasses the pulmonary circuitry
- Growth problems and relative anemia can be caused by increased oxygen consumption and decreased nutrient intake
- Increased infections are seen in conjunction with associated syndromes such as asplenia or DiGeorge syndrome (congenital absence of the thymus)

TABLE 17-1 Summary of classic findings in CHD

Lesion	PE findings	CXR	ECG	Rx
TOF	+/– murmur Single S2 and right ventricular heave	"Boot-shaped heart" (due to small pulmonary artery)	RVH +/– RAE	PGE1
Tricuspid atresia	+/– murmur Single S2	Normal size Decreased pulmonary markings	LAD RAE (older patients)	PGE1
Pulmonic atresia	+/– murmur Single S2	Cardiomegaly (due to LVH or RAE)	LAD LVH RAE	PGE1
TGA	+/– murmur	"Egg on a string" (due to A/P positioning of the aorta and pulmonary artery)	Normal	PGE1
TAPVR + obstruction	Widely split S2	Congestive heart failure	RAD RVH RAE	Lasix Digoxin
Truncus arteriosus	Wide pulse pressures + murmur across single valve	Cardiomegaly Congestive heart failure +/– Absence of thymus (association with DiGeorge syndrome)	Biventricular hypertrophy	Lasix Digoxin
Aortic coarctation	Delayed or weak femoral pulses Harsh systolic murmur in left axilla and back	Normal early in life	RVH (neonatal) LVH (later presentation)	PGE1

PE, physical examination; Rx, drug-medication LAD, left axis deviation; RAD, right axis deviation; A-P, anterior-posterior.

Lesions with Decreased Pulmonary Blood Flow

Tetralogy of Fallot (TOF) is the most common form of CCHD in children who present outside of the newborn period. Patients with TOF have the following four defects (see Figure 17-1), (a) An aorta that overrides the VSD, (b) Right ventricular outflow tract obstruction, (c) Large unrestrictive VSD, and (d) RVH. The degree of outflow tract obstruction varies, and therefore the age of presentation and severity at time of presentation can vary considerably. Infants with very severe obstruction from birth present with cyanosis in the first several days of life as the ductus arteriosus closes. These infants require prostaglandin-E1 (PGE1) to maintain the patency of the ductus in order to survive. Infants born with less severe outflow tract obstruction will present later, usually within the first several years of life as the obstruction progresses. They often have "tet" spells, as described in the discussion in the opening vignette. Treatment is surgical and begins with the Blalock-Taussig shunt (see Box 17-7). Definitive correction involves closure of the VSD with augmentation of the right ventricular outflow tract.

Tricuspid atresia is characterized by the complete absence of the tricuspid valve and a hypoplastic

right ventricle. It is always associated with a VSD. All systemic flow travels across the patent foramen ovale (which remains patent due to elevated RA pressures) and into the left side of the heart. When the VSD is large, there may not be any compromise to the pulmonary circulation at all, as blood will flow freely from the

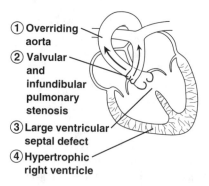

① **Overriding aorta**
② **Valvular and infundibular pulmonary stenosis**
③ **Large ventricular septal defect**
④ **Hypertrophic right ventricle**

FIGURE 17-1   Four classic anatomic features of tetralogy of Fallot. (1) Overriding aorta (dextroposition of the aorta). (2) Obstruction to right ventricular outflow (infundibular or valvular pulmonic stenosis). (3) Ventricular septal defect. (4) Right ventricular hypertrophy. (From Blackbourne LH, *Advanced Surgical Recall*, 2nd ed. Baltimore: Lippincott Williams & Wilkins, 2004.)

Definitive surgical correction in patients with congenital cardiac anomalies is performed to reestablish "normal" circulation patterns, but these procedures are often unsafe or technically impossible in very young patients. Shunt procedures are therefore often performed in patients with decreased blood flow to the lungs prior to definitive correction as temporizing measures which allow for increased mixing of oxygenated and deoxygenated blood thereby improving systemic oxygenation and resulting in improved growth and development. Shunts that increase blood flow to the lungs also help retard the development of pulmonary hypertension, which will adversely affect long-term survival.

The Blalock-Taussig (B-T) shunt, which creates an anastomosis between the right subclavian artery and the ipsilateral pulmonary artery, is the most common shunt performed. This in effect provides blood flow to the lungs, albeit systemic blood (i.e., blood pumped into the aorta by the left ventricle). In the classic B-T shunt, the subclavian artery was ligated and reanastomosed with the right pulmonary artery, thus sacrificing the subclavian artery for this procedure. The modified B-T shunt, which is the most common technique used today, uses a Gore-tex conduit between the subclavian and pulmonary artery and thus spares the subclavian artery. B-T shunts are used most commonly to reestablish pulmonary blood flow in children with either severe stenosis or atresia of the tricuspid or pulmonic valves.

tricuspid regurgitation murmur can be appreciated at the left lower sternal border. Chest x-ray reveals decreased pulmonary vasculature and possible cardiomegaly due to LVH or RAE. ECG similarly demonstrates left axis deviation and LVH with RAE. Immediate management involves PGE1 continuous infusion, otherwise cyanosis progresses rapidly and the infant will die. A Blalock-Taussig shunt is necessary to increase pulmonary blood flow. Further surgical intervention is dependent on the degree of RVH. If the ventricle is severely compromised, then a Fontan procedure is performed.

Lesions with Increased Pulmonary Blood Flow

Total anomalous pulmonary venous return (TAPVR) represents an embryologic failure in connecting the pulmonary vein and the left atrium (see Figure 17-2). Instead, one of several embryologic connections is maintained between the pulmonary vein and the blood flow into the right side of the heart. This aberrant connection can be between the pulmonary vein and the superior vena cava (SVC) (supracardiac), the portal venous system (infracardiac), or into the RA via the coronary sinus. When pulmonary venous flow to any of these three sites is compromised, it is referred to as *TAPVR with obstruction* and these are the infants who present early in the newborn period with cyanosis and respiratory distress. Pulmonary edema

left ventricle into the pulmonary artery. However, in cases with smaller VSDs or over time as the VSD tends to decrease in size, pulmonary flow will decrease. Age at presentation is dependent on the size of the VSD. Infants with very small VSDs, and who are therefore dependent on the ductus arteriosus for pulmonary blood flow, will present as neonates when the ductus closes. For patients who present in the neonatal period, PGE1 is essential. Surgical intervention involves first the placement of a temporizing Blalock-Taussig shunt. The subsequent corrective surgery is known as a modified Fontan and involves a staged procedure that ultimately connects the superior vena cava directly to the pulmonary artery, bypassing the right side of the heart.

Pulmonic atresia with intact ventricular septum is associated with varying degrees of a hypoplastic right ventricle. It is always associated with an ASD with blood flow from right to left. Pulmonary blood flow is dependent on the ductus arteriosus and, therefore, these rare patients present very early in the neonatal period as the ductus closes. Physical examination reveals a single S_2 heart sound and sometimes a

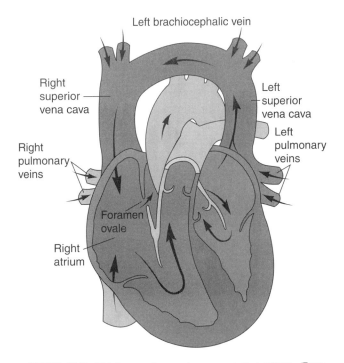

FIGURE 17-2   Total anomalous pulmonary venous return. (From Pillitteri, A. *Maternal and Child Nursing,* 4th ed., Philadelphia: Lippincott Williams & Wilkins, 2003.)

develops from the obstructed pulmonary venous out-flow and this manifests itself with progressive respiratory distress. Cyanosis also develops due to the decreased volume of oxygenated blood returning to the RA. PGE1 administration is *contraindicated* in patients with TAPVR with obstruction as it will only further increase pulmonary congestion by increasing blood flow to the lungs via the ductus. Lasix is useful to help decrease the pulmonary congestion and digoxin is often used when a significant component of heart failure is present. In cases with severe obstruction, surgery is necessary, often within the first month of life. Surgical correction creates a wide connection between the common pulmonary vein and the posterior wall of the left atrium, allowing for oxygenated blood to drain directly into the left atrium.

In patients with *Truncus arteriosus* (TA), the aorta, pulmonary artery, and coronary arteries all arise from a single trunk at the base of the heart with a single semilunar valve and an obligatory VSD (see Figure 17-3). This configuration allows for mixing of oxygenated and deoxygenated blood and therefore the oxygen content of the systemic circulation is roughly equal to that of the pulmonary artery. In the weeks following birth as the pulmonary vascular resistance drops, blood flow to the lungs increases and signs and symptoms of heart failure will soon develop from volume overload. When pulmonary overload occurs, then pulmonary vascular resistance again rises and biventricular hypertrophy results from the strain on both ventricles. Medical therapy is aimed at treating the heart failure and uses diuretics and digoxin. Surgical

correction involves closure of the VSD so that the truncus is enclosed within the left ventricle only. Subsequently, the pulmonary artery is removed from the posterior portion of the aorta and a conduit is used to connect it with the right ventricle.

Transposition of the great arteries (TGA) is another form of CCHD, and is in fact the most common lesion seen in cyanotic infants who present in the newborn period. TGA can be associated with an ASD or VSD and in such cases, it is referred to as complex TGA. The most common form, however, is an isolated anomaly without additional cardiac defects. In isolated TGA, the pulmonary and systemic circulations work in parallel rather than in series. Thus, the only path which allows for mixing of oxygenated and deoxygenated blood is the ductus arteriosus. Cyanosis is typically present at birth due to the mixing of oxygenated blood from the pulmonary artery and deoxygenated blood from the aorta via the ductus. Cyanosis progresses as the ductus closes. Severe hypoxemia, acidosis, and death can occur rapidly.

Children diagnosed with TGA should be started on a PGE1 infusion immediately as it is lifesaving. More definitive treatment involves perforation of the fossa ovalis with a balloon catheter in an effort to improve mixing. More definitive surgical correction involves switching the circulations at the level of the great vessels. They are divided at the level of the aortic and pulmonic valves and then switched so that the aortic valve, which arises from the right ventricle, is connected to the pulmonary artery and the pulmonary valve, which arises from the left ventricle, is connected to the aorta.

Acyanotic Congenital Heart Disease

Acyanotic conditions involve cardiac lesions that result in left-to-right shunting and therefore allow for normal arterial oxygen saturation. Examples of such cardiac defects include ASDs, VSDs, patent ductus arteriosus (PDAs), and endocardial cushion defects (also known as atrioventricular [AV] canal defects). The main consequence of such lesions is that pulmonary blood flow is increased due to the shunting of blood to the right side of the heart, and over time pulmonary hypertension will develop and may ultimately increase to a point that pulmonary pressures rise to systemic pressures or above. In this case, the shunt would reverse and become right-to-left and the resulting physiology would then approximate that of the previously discussed cyanotic lesions, which collectively result in decreased arterial oxygen saturation. A second set of congenital cardiac lesions which result in normal oxygen saturation but decreased systemic blood flow are those which are isolated obstructive lesions, such as coarctation of the aorta.

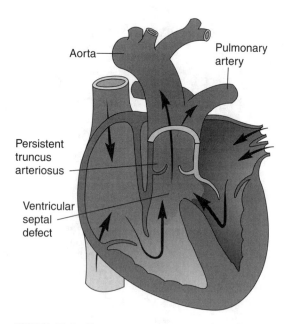

FIGURE 17-3 Truncus arteriosus. (From Pillitteri, A., *Maternal and Child Nursing*, 4th ed., Philadelphia: Lippincott Williams & Wilkins, 2003.)

Aortic coarctation describes a condition in which there is congenital narrowing of the aorta. Simple coarctation is defined as coarctation without any other associated cardiac lesions and occurs most often at the level of the ductus arteriosus just distal to the branching of the left subclavian artery (see Figure 17-4). When the ductus arteriosus is open early in the neonatal period, blood can bypass the obstruction via the ductus and therefore reach systemic circulation. However, when the ductus closes, systemic circulation will be indirectly proportional to the degree of narrowing. In most cases there is decreased but sufficient blood flow leading to a diagnosis later in life. However, in cases where the narrowing is severe, systemic circulation will be significantly compromised and patients present with signs and symptoms of shock in the first several weeks of life. The hallmark of aortic coarctation is increased blood pressures in the upper extremities compared to the lower extremities with femoral pulses which are weak and/or delayed.

For the small subset of patients with severe aortic coarctation, medical management is required urgently as the ductus closes. Surgical correction is often performed urgently following initial stabilization, which involves the administration of PGE1 to open the ductus in addition to inotropic medications such as digitalis that improve the contractility of the heart and its ability to work against the obstruction. There are many surgical procedures for correction of aortic coarctation, yet most commonly the stenotic area of

the aorta is resected and a direct end-to-end anastomosis if performed.

KEY POINTS

- When an infant presents in shock in the first 1 to 2 weeks of life think:
  - Sepsis
  - CHD
  - Adrenal dysfunction
- When CHD is suspected, early prostaglandin administration can be lifesaving!
  - PGE1 has little downside
  - Not beneficial in TAPVR or TA but also not particularly harmful
  - Consider intubation before administering because of apnea
- Central cyanosis is always pathologic
  - Involves mucous membranes and lips
  - Acrocyanosis is benign and involves only hands and feet
- Cardiac murmurs important in evaluating cyanotic child
  - Physiologic murmurs are soft, short, and in early systole
  - Pathologic murmurs are loud, longer, and in various parts of the cardiac cycle
- Use oxygen with caution in cyanotic newborns
  - Acceleration of ductus arteriosus closure may worsen condition
  - Oxygen may not increase PaO_2 in many cardiac lesions
  - Administer oxygen to maintain oxygen saturation greater than 75%
- Cardiac anomalies that result in increased pulmonary blood flow, left-to-right shunting
  - TGA
  - TAPVR (with or without obstruction)
  - TA
  - Treatment involves Lasix and digoxin +/− PGE1
- Cardiac anomalies that result in decreased pulmonary blood flow, right-to-left shunting
  - TOF
  - Tricuspid atresia
- Temporizing surgery is a Blalock-Taussig shunt
  - Provides pulmonary blood flow from systemic circulation
  - In effect acts as the ductus arteriosus with left-to-right shunting

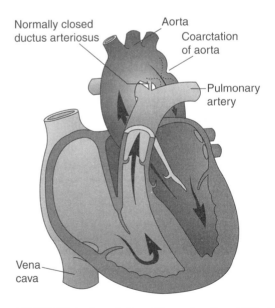

FIGURE 17-4   Coarctation of the aorta. (From Pillitteri, A. *Maternal and Child Nursing*, 4th ed., Philadelphia: Lippincott Williams & Wilkins, 2003.)

CHAPTER 18

Neonatal Jaundice—Indirect Hyperbilirubinemia

CASE SCENARIO

A 4-day-old Asian boy presents to the ED in his mother's arms. She reports that he is "yellow" and has not been feeding well over the past 24 hours. He was born at 42 weeks' gestation via vaginal delivery with vacuum-assisted extraction. Initially, he fed vigorously, yet over the last day he has not been waking to feed as often and has been wetting his diapers less frequently. His vital signs on admission to the ED are a rectal temperature 98.2°F, pulse of 166, blood pressure of 60/40, and a respiratory rate of 48. The physical examination reveals a newborn who is sleeping but wakes and cries with the examination. You find a large occipital cephalohematoma and note jaundice to the level of his knees. His skin turgor is good. The remainder of his examination is unremarkable.

1. Which of the factors in his history does not place him at additional risk for development of hyperbilirubinemia?
   a. Asian male
   b. Late gestational age
   c. Cephalohematoma
   d. Exclusively breast-fed

East Asian race, the presence of cephalohematomas, and exclusive breastfeeding are several risk factors for the development of severe hyperbilirubinemia. Premature infants < 37 weeks gestational age are much more at risk for developing hyperbilirubinemia than are full-term infants (37 to 42 weeks). Infants born at gestational age > 41 weeks are actually associated with a decreased risk of significant jaundice.

2. What is a critical piece of the history that must be elicited very early in this patient's assessment?
   a. The mother's blood type
   b. Family history of hyperbilirubinemia
   c. Risk factors for neonatal sepsis
   d. Stooling pattern

Neonatal sepsis can present with poor feeding and jaundice; therefore, it is paramount that the patient's risk for sepsis be elucidated upon presentation. The patient's mother informs you that she had excellent prenatal care and that neither she nor the baby received antibiotics in the peripartum period. They were both discharged from the hospital in 48 hours. He has had neither high nor low temperatures at home. Based on this patient's examination and risk for severe hyperbilirubinemia, but low risk for sepsis, you order a total serum bilirubin which is elevated to 21.8 mg/dL.

3. Which additional laboratory test is most important to obtain prior to the start of phototherapy treatment?
   a. Hematocrit with reticulocyte count
   b. Infant's blood type
   c. Direct antibody testing
   d. Direct bilirubin

The hematocrit, reticulocyte count, blood type, and indirect and direct antibody testing will provide useful information regarding this patient's etiology of hyperbilirubinemia and the extent to which hemolysis is occurring secondary to ABO incompatibility.

However, regardless of etiology, this patient meets requirements for treatment of hyperbilirubinemia and should be admitted for phototherapy treatment. Prior to starting phototherapy, it should be documented that this patient does not have direct hyperbilirubinemia, because phototherapy is not useful in this setting and, in fact, can result in long-term pigmentation of the skin. You obtain a direct bilirubin level that is normal at 1.8 mg/dL. You also obtain the infant's and mother's blood types, with antibody testing, which reveals no indication for ABO or Rh incompatibility.

Answers: 1-b, 2-c, 3-d

DEFINITION

Neonatal jaundice is a very common condition, occurring in > 50% of newborns. It does not often require medical therapy, nor is it frequently associated with any long-term sequelae. Rarely, however, severely elevated bilirubin levels can be associated with bilirubin encephalopathy and kernicterus with associated neurodevelopmental devastation. Hyperbilirubinemia in the first 24 hours of life, or in infants 2 weeks or older, is always considered pathologic and its etiology must be evaluated and treated. Physical evidence of jaundice is seen when the bilirubin levels reach 5 to 10 mg/dL. Jaundice progresses in a head-to-toe fashion and bilirubin estimates can be made based on the extent of jaundice (9, nipples; 12, groin; 15, knees; and >15, below the knees), although these estimates are often inaccurate and should not be replaced by laboratory confirmation if treatment for hyperbilirubinemia is in question.

ETIOLOGY

Physiologic Jaundice of the Newborn

Normal physiology of the newborn is often the cause of neonatal jaundice, and therefore it is often referred to as *physiologic jaundice of the newborn.* Infants are born with an increased red blood cell (RBC) mass and shortened RBC survival; therefore, they have increased hemolysis and bilirubin production. Hepatic immaturity results in decreased levels of glucuronyl transferase, an enzyme necessary for bilirubin conjugation and its subsequent excretion. Physiologic jaundice begins on the second to fourth day of life, often peaks by the third to fifth days, and resolves within 1 to 2 weeks. Physiologic jaundice is a diagnosis of exclusion and more serious reasons for neonatal jaundice must be considered.

Hemolytic Jaundice

Hemolysis should be the first consideration in the setting of indirect (unconjugated) hyperbilirubinemia. The most frequent hemolytic condition is ABO incompatibility. Rh isoimmunization can also be responsible, although less frequently. Red cell enzyme defects such as glucose-6-phosphate dehydrogenase (G6PD) deficiency and membrane disorders such as hereditary spherocytosis can lead to hemolytic jaundice. These conditions are more common in certain ethnic backgrounds such as Mediterranean and northern European, respectively. If hemolytic disease is suspected, ABO blood typing of the mother and infant should be obtained, as well as an RBC smear to look for schistocytes. A complete blood count (CBC) should also be obtained to assess the severity of anemia and to look for an elevated reticulocyte count, which suggests hemolysis.

Nonhemolytic Jaundice

In the absence of hemolysis, physiologic jaundice is the most common etiology of neonatal indirect hyperbilirubinemia. Other nonhemolytic causes include "breast milk jaundice," which is thought to be due to the presence of glucuronyl transferase inhibitor in breast milk, resulting in a prolonged unconjugated hyperbilirubinemia. Breast milk jaundice typically occurs after the first 4 to 7 days of life. This should be differentiated from "breast-feeding jaundice," which occurs before the first 4 to 7 days of life and is caused by insufficient production or intake of breast milk and a relative dehydration with decreased plasma volume and subsequent increased concentrations of bilirubin. Breast-feeding jaundice is often considered an exaggerated state of physiologic jaundice since there is increased enterohepatic circulation, decreased stooling, and decreased bilirubin excretion. Other etiologies of nonhemolytic jaundice include internal hemorrhage, most commonly seen

---

BOX 18-1   Indications for hospitalization in hyperbilirubinemia

- Gestational age < 37 weeks
- Blood group incompatibility: ABO, Rh, Kell, and Duffy
- Infection
- Polycythemia
- Hematomas or excessive bruising
- Infant of diabetic mother
- Hypoalbuminemia
- Red blood cell membrane or enzyme defects (G6PD deficiency, hereditary spherocytosis, pyruvate kinase deficiency)
- Hemoglobinopathies
- Crigler-Najjar disease

---

as cephalohematomas or less often as subdural hematomas. Infants born with polycythemia or to a diabetic mother are also at increased risk of developing indirect hyperbilirubinemia (see Box 18-1).

Although it is rare for infections or neonatal sepsis to present with jaundice as the only symptom, it is very important to rule out an infectious etiology for neonatal jaundice by history and physical examination. Doing a full sepsis workup will depend on other factors such as fever, feeding, vomiting, and overall appearance. A sepsis workup is indicated in newborns who become jaundiced within 24 hours of birth.

A Word about Neonatal Direct Hyperbilirubinemia

As mentioned previously, a vast majority of jaundice in the newborns is caused by increased levels of indirect bilirubin. However, a small number of newborns can have jaundice secondary to direct hyperbilirubinemia, which is defined as a direct bilirubin level that exceeds 20% of the total bilirubin value. These infants usually present to their primary care provider or to the ED with prolonged jaundice and abnormally light stools or dark urine. There are many causes of direct hyperbilirubinemia in newborns, yet the majority of cases are caused by only a few etiologies. In a newborn who is not total parenteral nutrition (TPN) dependent, these etiologies include extrahepatic biliary atresia, neonatal hepatitis (idiopathic and infectious), alpha-1-antitrypsin deficiency, and Alagille syndrome. Conditions such as sepsis, hypothyroidism, panhypopituitarism, and inborn errors of metabolism should also be considered.

TREATMENT

Therapy for indirect hyperbilirubinemia depends on the age of the patient and the total serum bilirubin (TSB) level. Phototherapy is the first-line treatment

for hyperbilirubinemia. On rare occasions, exchange transfusion is indicated for extreme TSB levels (often > 25 mg/dL) or if signs of the intermediate to advanced stages of acute bilirubin encephalopathy exist (hypertonia, arching, retrocollis, opisthotonos, fever, high-pitched cry). In general, the treatment threshold is dependent on the infant's age in hours and is not an absolute number. Rather, it is a stratified risk based on the gestational age and the presence of risk factors for the development of severe hyperbilirubinemia. The Bhutani curve (see Figure 18-1) depicts three lines based on risk factors that define the treatment threshold given age. If the TSB level falls above the line for a given age, then treatment should be administered. This graph can also be used to plot TSB levels over several days. Treatment may be initiated in infants with a steep upward trajectory (i.e., crossing percentile lines) even though the absolute TSB level has not yet reached the threshold.

For example, the 4-year-old boy in the opening case scenario who is approximately 96 hours old, without identifiable risk factors for sepsis, well-appearing, and a TSB of 22 mg/dL, has a treatment threshold of approximately 20 mg/dL. He should therefore be admitted for phototherapy since his level surpasses the threshold. In addition, the question of rehydration should be addressed. Often supplementation of formula for a day or two while continuing to breast-feed will rehydrate infants

---

LITERATURE REFERENCE

 Should Sn-mesoporphyrin be used as an adjunct to phototherapy?

Martinez et al. looked at tin-mesoporphyrin (SnMP), a potent inhibitor of bilirubin production, and evaluated its role in (a) moderating the need for phototherapy in full-term breast-fed infants with plasma bilirubin concentrations ≥ 15 mg/dL and ≤ 18 mg/dL that were reached between ≥ 48 and ≤ 96 hours of age, (b) diminishing the time required for the plasma bilirubin concentration to decline to ≤ 13 mg/dL, and (c) decreasing the number of bilirubin determinations required for monitoring hyperbilirubinemia. They found that a single dose of SnMP proved effective in all of these measures. SnMP does not yet have FDA approval for use in the United States [**Martinez JC et al. *Pediatrics* 1999;103:1–5**].

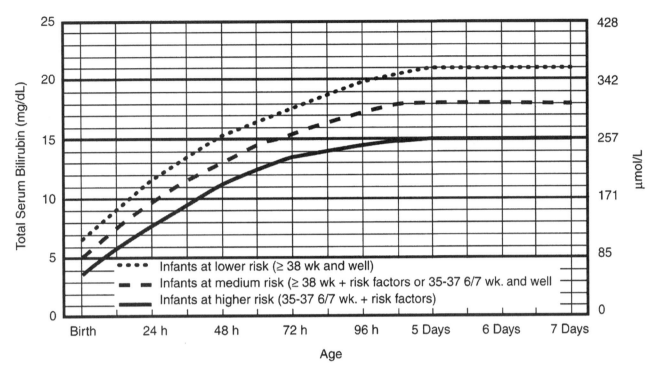

- Use total bilirubin. Do not subtract direct reacting or conjugated bilirubin.
- Risk factors = isoimmune hemolytic disease, G6PD deficiency, asphyxia, significant lethargy, temperature instability, sepsis, acidosis, or albumin < 3.0g/dL (if measured).
- For well infants 35-37 6/7 wk can adjust TSB levels for intervention around the medium risk line. It is an option to intervene at lower TSB levels for infants closer to 35 wk and at higher TSB levels for those closer to 37 6/7 wk.
- It is an option to provide conventional phototherapy in hospital or at home at TSB levels 2-3 mg/dL (35-50 mmol/L) below those shown but home phototherapy should not be used in any infant with risk factors.

FIGURE 18-1   Bhutani curve. (From American Academy of Pediatrics from the Subcommittee on Hyperbilirubinemia. Management of hyperbilirubinemia in the newborn Infant 35 or more weeks of gestation. *Pediatrics.* July 2004;114(1):297–316 with permission.)

and increase the excretion of bilirubin. Some families are averse to supplementation, and the need for IV hydration versus continued breastfeeding with close monitoring of hydration status must be weighed.

KEY POINTS

- Hyperbilirubinemia in neonates is most often indirect
- Jaundice in a neonate < 24-hours-old is always pathologic
  - Sepsis workup necessary
- Jaundice in a neonate between days 2 and 7 of life is most often physiologic
  - Exaggerated when seen in the context of breast-feeding—"breast-feeding jaundice"
  - Sepsis workup not necessary unless fever, ill-appearing, vomiting, etc.

- Hemolytic conditions can exaggerate physiologic neonatal jaundice
  - Often produce more severe hyperbilirubinemia
  - Most common example is ABO incompatibility
- Bhutani curve gives threshold TSB level for treatment based on age and risk factors
- Phototherapy is most commonly used to treat hyperbilirubinemia
- Exchange transfusion may be required in severe forms

CHAPTER 19

Malrotation

CASE SCENARIO

On a busy night in the ED, you receive a call from the triage nurse at the front desk. She has just registered a 3-week-old newborn who has been vomiting, but is otherwise reported to be well appearing.

1. Which of the following piece of information would compel you to see this patient immediately?
   a. Rectal temperature of 101°F
   b. Bilious emesis
   c. Guaiac positive diarrhea
   d. Blood pressure of 65/38

Bilious emesis in an infant should be considered an emergency. Malrotation with an associated midgut volvulus should be suspected until proven otherwise. Evaluation and treatment should be immediate, as these children can decompensate extremely quickly from relatively well-appearing to near-death within a matter of 1 hour as bowel ischemia ensues. Fever in the newborn also requires prompt attention; however, unlike bilious emesis it can wait for a few minutes in an otherwise well appearing infant. Of course, it is necessary to take a quick look at the child before delaying evaluation to make sure that he/she is in fact well appearing. Guaiac positive diarrhea has numerous etiologies, ranging from viral gastroenteritis to milk protein allergy to intussusception. Patients with malrotation and volvulus may have guaiac positive stools as well, yet it would be extremely rare for these patients to present without bilious emesis. A blood pressure of 65/38 is within normal limits for an infant of this age, and therefore should not be cause for alarm. Hypotension for term infants, according to Pediatric Advanced Life Support (PALS) guidelines 2002, is defined as a systolic blood pressure (SBP) less than 60 mm Hg.

Given this history, you evaluate the infant in triage. She is with her mother, yet she is irritable and somewhat inconsolable. Her abdomen is soft and nondistended. Her pulse is slightly elevated at 180 beats per minute (bpm). She is warm and well-perfused. You repeat her blood pressure and it is stable at 68/40. You notice her mother's shirt is stained bright green with the baby's vomit.

2. What is the next step in this infant's management?
   a. Place an IV and initiate a 20 cc/kg bolus of normal saline (NS)
   b. Place a nasogastric (NG) tube to decompress the stomach
   c. Observe the child until she vomits again to determine bile content
   d. Call for surgical consultation

This child requires immediate resuscitation given that she is inconsolable and the apparent bile on the mother's shirt. Parents often mistake yellow-tinged emesis as bilious. However, true bilious emesis is green, not yellow. Gastric secretions themselves are yellow and can often be misinterpreted as bile. Obviously, one does not need to directly visualize green emesis to take the complaint seriously, yet because there can be confusion surrounding this descriptive term, it is important to elicit from the parents exactly what they mean by "bilious" emesis.

Resuscitation should begin with IV access and a NS bolus. Laboratory tests should include a complete blood count (CBC), electrolytes, liver function tests, and lipase. Blood cultures should also be sent. While this is being done, both surgery and radiology should be notified.

3. What is the best radiologic study to order in an infant suspected of having malrotation with volvulus?
   a. Kidney, ureter, and bladder (KUB) plain film
   b. Computed tomography (CT) scan
   c. Abdominal ultrasound
   d. Upper gastrointestinal contrast study (UGI)

Abdominal plain films vary considerably in patients with midgut volvulus. They may be nonspecific, or they may reveal evidence of obstruction including marked gastric and duodenal dilatation with a paucity of gas distally. The most reliable study in the diagnosis of malrotation with or without volvulus is the UGI. Ultrasonography can be suggestive of malrotation if it reveals inversion of the superior mesenteric artery and vein. A CT scan will also show malrotation; however, it is not usually used when entertaining this diagnosis because a UGI is much quicker.

You initiate a 20 cc/kg bolus of NS and place an NG tube for the administration of contrast for the study. You accompany the infant for her UGI, which reveals malposition of the ligament of Treitz and a "corkscrew" appearance as the contrast travels through the duodenum. These findings confirm the diagnosis of malrotation. You return with the patient to the ED and she continues to appear well. Thirty minutes later the nurse informs you that the infant's pulse has climbed to 210 and her blood pressure has fallen to 55/40. When you examine the child, you note that she is slightly mottled with a distended and firm abdomen.

4. What is the next step in her management?
   a. Repeat 20 cc/kg bolus of NS
   b. Start broad-coverage IV antibiotics
   c. Initiate vasopressor therapy to increase cardiac output
   d. Call the operating room (OR) for emergent surgery

This infant has midgut volvulus with resulting ischemic bowel, which is rapidly fatal. The only priority at this point is getting the infant to the OR. While this is being arranged, a repeat bolus of NS is given. Broad-coverage antibiotics are administered as well (ampicillin 50 mg/kg, gentamicin 4 mg/kg, and metronidazole (Flagyl) 15 mg/kg). Vasopressors may be necessary if the infant does not respond to the fluid bolus. An exploratory laparotomy performed in the OR reveals torsed small intestine that appears deep purple and edematous. This section of intestine is resected and a reanastomosis is performed. The child is stabilized postoperatively in the surgical intensive care unit (SICU).

Answers: 1-b, 2-a, 3-d, 4-d

DEFINITION

Intestinal malrotation is defined as the incomplete rotation and abnormal fixation of the gut during embryologic development. Because the intestine is not properly fixated, it is at risk for twisting on its own blood supply, a condition known as volvulus. The incidence of malrotation in the United States is estimated at 1 in 500 live births. Seventy-five percent of patients with malrotation will develop a volvulus, and 75% of these will present within the first month of life. The remainder of cases can present any time in life and may be discovered incidentally during other procedures, or even at autopsy. When a volvulus occurs at the site of the malrotated small intestine it is termed midgut volvulus. In neonates, malrotation with midgut volvulus is twice as common in boys as girls. After age 1, there is no gender predilection. Malrotation is often associated with several other congenital anomalies of the abdominal wall, gut, heart, or spleen (see Box 19-1.)

ETIOLOGY

In normal development, the intestinal tract begins as a straight tube from stomach to rectum. Between the fourth and eighth weeks of gestation, the majority of the developing gut (distal duodenum to transverse colon) leaves the abdominal cavity and enters the umbilical cord progressively as it grows. By the 10th week of gestation, this protruding portion of bowel

Gastrointestinal
- Congenital diaphragmatic hernia
- Abdominal wall defects
  - Omphalocele
  - Gastroschisis
  - Prune belly syndrome
- Atresias
  - Duodenal
  - Jejunoileal
  - Esophageal +/– tracheoesophageal fistula
  - Biliary
- Meckel's diverticulum
- Duodenal web or stenosis
- Hirschsprung disease
- Imperforate anus

Other
- Trisomies
  - Chromosomes 8, 13, and 21
- Congenital cardiac defects
- Heterotaxy syndromes
  - Polysplenia
  - Asplenia

returns to the fetal abdominal cavity. Under normal circumstances, the bowel returns and rotates a total of 270 degrees using the superior mesenteric artery (SMA) as its axis thereby transitioning itself from a vertical plane (as it was in the umbilicus) to a horizontal plane. The duodenojejunal loop rotates to the region of the ligament of Treitz and becomes fixed to the posterior peritoneum. The portion of colon which has herniated into the umbilicus also returns to the abdominal cavity and enters the left upper quadrant. This portion also becomes fixed to the posterior abdominal wall. When the cecum reenters the abdomen, it rotates in a counterclockwise motion and settles in the right lower quadrant. Reversal or arrest of any of these multiple stages of gut development can result in malpositioned and unfixated portions of bowel, and is responsible for the range of anomalies and clinical presentations seen.

The most common anomaly is complete nonrotation of the midgut. This occurs when the duodenojejunal limb and the cecocolic limbs fail to rotate upon re-entry into the abdominal cavity. As a result, there is no duodenal loop from the right to left side of the abdomen. This results in the ligament of Treitz being located on the right side of the abdomen. Similarly, the cecum ends up in the left side of the abdomen. In nonrotation, the proximal jejunum and ascending colon are fused together as one pedicle,

through which the blood supply (SMA) to the entire midgut is located. This portion of bowel acts as the pedicle on which a midgut volvulus occurs, leading to ischemic necrosis of the entire midgut.

CLINICAL PRESENTATION

Presentation varies according to the type of defect and also with the duration of symptoms. Malrotation without volvulus often has a very insidious and chronic presentation, characterized by intermittent abdominal pain with or without emesis, diarrhea, and/or constipation. Malrotation in an infant can be initially misdiagnosed as colic. Recurrent mild symptoms are likely due to transient twisting of the bowel. Partial blockage of the venous and lymphatic drainage can cause problems with nutrient absorption and protein loss, leading to failure to thrive. Many children with malrotation never develop symptoms, as is the case in half of adolescents with malrotation.

Malrotation with midgut volvulus presents much more acutely and is characterized by symptoms of acute intestinal obstruction (e.g., abdominal pain and bilious emesis). The obstruction in midgut volvulus is usually proximal, and therefore abdominal distention is often absent in the early stages. When the diagnosis is delayed, symptoms can progress rapidly. The abdomen becomes markedly distended and tender with peritoneal signs as the bowel wall infarction occurs. Severe dehydration, shock, and death ensue rapidly if not treated properly (see Box 19-2).

DIAGNOSIS

Plain films, ultrasound, and UGI have all been used in the diagnosis of malrotation and midgut volvulus. UGI is considered the gold standard of diagnosis. The classic finding is a corkscrew appearance as the contrast winds through twisted bowel or a "bird's

- Malrotation +/– midgut volvulus
- Duodenal atresia
- Intussusception
- Incarcerated hernias
- Meconium ileus
- Hirschsprung disease
- Necrotizing enterocolitis
- Sepsis
- Congenital adrenal hyperplasia

beak" as the contrast tapers and then stops at the site of complete obstruction. This study will reveal the right-sided positioning of the small intestine which is diagnostic of malrotation, even in the absence of a midgut volvulus. Abdominal ultrasound can also be very sensitive in detecting malrotation with or without volvulus. Inversion of the superior mesenteric artery and vein suggests malrotation. Plain abdominal films are sometimes normal but may also show the classic "double bubble." This represents air in the stomach adjacent to air in the proximal portion of the duodenum caused by the distal obstruction. This finding would also suggest duodenal atresia, which typically presents in the first 24 to 48 hours of life. Keep in mind that diagnostic imaging is not necessary in an ill-appearing child with bilious emesis or with signs of peritonitis. These children should be taken emergently to the OR for exploratory laparotomy.

TREATMENT

Surgical intervention is the definitive treatment for malrotation and must be performed emergently when midgut volvulus is present. Initial resuscitation while surgery is being arranged includes aggressive fluid resuscitation (i.e., several boluses of NS as needed), broad-coverage IV antibiotics, and NG tube placement for stomach decompression. Operative management for most types of intestinal rotation anomalies is known as Ladd's procedure. This involves detorsion of the bowel, resection of any necrotic bowel, and lysis of Ladd's bands, which are fibrous tissue bands which extend from the cecum to the right upper quadrant and can often cause compression or obstruction of the duodenum. Any portion of bowel with questioned viability will often be left and re-evaluated intraoperatively within 24 to 48 hours in an attempt to avoid unnecessary bowel resection. The bowel is replaced in the abdominal cavity without pexy and with the entire small intestine on the right and the large intestine on the left. Consequently, an appendectomy is also performed because the appendix does not reside in the right lower quadrant, which could lead to delayed diagnosis if the child ever developed appendicitis in the future.

PROGNOSIS

The mortality rate for malrotation with midgut volvulus is between 3% and 25% depending on the delay to diagnosis and surgery. Mortality is higher for younger patients and those with associated anomalies. The most common complication following surgery is

short-gut syndrome, which leads to growth and nutritional problems. Recurrent volvulus is relatively infrequent but should be considered in any patient who develops obstructive symptoms in the postoperative period or thereafter.

KEY POINTS

- Bilious emesis in an infant should be considered a surgical emergency until proven otherwise
- Intestinal malrotation results from the incomplete rotation and abnormal fixation of the gut during embryologic development
- Midgut volvulus should be expected if bilious vomiting
  - Abdominal distention is usually absent due to the proximal location of the obstruction in the duodenum
  - Peritoneal signs are often late findings and indicative of bowel infarction
- More than 60% of patients with malrotation have associated anomalies
  - Polysplenia, asplenia, or congenital abdominal wall defects
  - Presence of these should lead to investigation for malrotation.
- UGI is the gold standard of diagnosis in a stable patient
  - Plain films or ultrasound are less sensitive alternatives
- Patients with suspected malrotation with midgut volvulus require aggressive resuscitation
  - IV NS in 20 cc/kg boluses
  - Broad-spectrum IV antibiotic
  - NG tube placement with gastric decompression
- Exploratory laparotomy with detorsion is the definitive treatment
  - Radiographic studies not necessary in an ill-appearing child with bilious emesis and peritonitis

CHAPTER 20

Pyloric Stenosis

CASE SCENARIO

A 6-week-old female infant arrives in the ED in the middle of the night, referred by her pediatrician for a 5-day history of progressive vomiting. The parents assume that most likely the vomiting is due to a "bug" as the patient's 3-year-old sibling has recently been diagnosed with rotavirus. They report that the baby was full term; she has been feeding and gaining weight very well until several days ago when she had some mild emesis, reported to be nonbloody and nonbilious. Since that time, they feel that the vomiting has increased in severity and now the baby is throwing up forcefully almost immediately after every bottle. They were surprised, however, that she continued to appear hungry and eager to feed almost all of the time until recently when she became sleepier and lost all interest in feeding. They note that she has had only one wet diaper in the past 12 hours and one normal stool. She has not had a fever. After soliciting this history, you begin to doubt that the patient has gastroenteritis, and instead suspect pyloric stenosis (PS).

1. Which of the following is not a risk factor for this condition?
   a. Female gender
   b. Age of 6 weeks
   c. Family history of the disease
   d. Breast-feeding

PS is at least four times more common in boys than in girls. PS is also more frequent in infants with affected siblings and children of affected mothers; and it is thought to be more frequent in infants who are breast-feeding.

You next review the patient's vital signs, which are significant for a normal temperature, blood pressure, and respiratory rate, and an elevated pulse of 180 beats per minute (bpm). The infant is sleepy but arousable; she has a slightly sunken anterior fontanelle, dry mucous membranes, and decreased skin turgor. Her heart and lung examinations are normal, with the exception of tachycardia. Her abdominal examination reveals a firm palpable mass just to the right of midline in the epigastric area, which heightens your suspicion for PS.

2. What is the next best step in her management?
   a. Place an IV and administer a normal saline (NS) bolus of 20 cc/kg
   b. Start IV ampicillin, gentamicin, and metronidazole (Flagyl)
   c. Administer oral rehydration solution (Pedialyte) through a nasogastric tube (NGT)
   d. Encourage breast-feeding

This patient's physical examination findings (tachycardia, sunken fontanelle, dry mucous membranes, and decreased skin turgor) suggest that she is approximately 10% dehydrated, which is considered severe. Your first priority should be to initiate proper fluid resuscitation. PS is not an infectious process and IV antibiotics are not indicated. While an NGT may be placed for comfort measures as it can be used to remove gastric secretions as they accumulate, it certainly should not be used for hydration purposes. Fluid delivered via an NGT will collect in the stomach and not be able to bypass the gastric outflow obstruction caused by the hypertrophied pylorus. For similar reasons, breast-feeding should be avoided once the diagnosis of PS is considered.

3. What is the best radiologic study to obtain in order to confirm the diagnosis?
   a. Kidney, ureter, and bladder (KUB) plain film
   b. Upper endoscopy
   c. Ultrasound
   d. Upper gastrointestinal contrast study (UGI)

Plain radiographs, such as a Supine and upright KUB, often are normal in PS. It is possible that a gasless abdomen and distended stomach will be visualized on KUB suggesting the diagnosis. UGI can reveal an elongated pyloric canal highly suggestive of PS, but this study increases the risk of vomiting and aspiration. Ultrasound is noninvasive and does not expose the child to radiation. It is the test of choice, provided an experienced ultrasonographer is available. You obtain an abdominal ultrasound that shows an epigastric mass suspicious for PS and you page a pediatric surgeon to come see the patient. In the meantime, the patient's laboratory values return.

4. Which results would be most consistent with PS?
    a. Hypokalemic, hyperchloremic metabolic acidosis
    b. Hyperkalemic, hyperchloremic metabolic acidosis
    c. Hypokalemic, hypochloremic metabolic alkalosis
    d. Hyperkalemic, hypochloremic metabolic alkalosis

Repeated vomiting produces a hypochloremic metabolic alkalosis due to the loss of hydrogen and chloride ions in the vomitus. In an effort to compensate for the alkalosis, intracellular hydrogen ions shift outside the cells in exchange for potassium ions, producing a relative hypokalemia. The patient's laboratory tests reveal a potassium of 3 mEq/dL, a chloride of 92 mEq/dL, and a bicarbonate of 34 mEq/dL. You talk with the surgeon who is in the operating room (OR) and unable to see the patient for another 2 hours.

5. What is the next best step in this patient's management?
    a. Transfer the patient to another facility for immediate surgical correction
    b. Administer a second NS bolus of 20 cc/kg
    c. Restart oral hydration
    d. Administer IV potassium 1 mEq/kg.

In infants with PS, medical resuscitation takes precedence over immediate surgical intervention. Severe dehydration and potential electrolyte imbalances are the most urgent issues and must be corrected prior to surgery. This child should be kept non per os (NPO) and receive a second NS bolus based on her severe dehydration. Hypokalemia will often correct with fluid resuscitation and should not be replenished in this case.

Answers: 1-a, 2-a, 3-c, 4-c, 5-b

DEFINITION

Pylorics stenosis (PS), also known as infantile hypertrophic pyloric stenosis (IHPS), is caused by hypertrophy of the muscular layers of the pylorus of the stomach. This is a progressive process, which ultimately can lead to total obstruction of the gastric outlet. In fact, this condition is the most common cause of intestinal obstruction in infancy. It occurs in approximately 3 in 1,000 live births and is at least four times more common in boys than girls and more common in whites than Hispanics or African-Americans. The age range of presentation is between 3 weeks and 5 months, yet most commonly PS presents at about 1 month of life.

The Hungry Vomiter

Infants with PS are described as "hungry vomiters," meaning that they often have episodes of forceful or "projectile" vomiting and then want to feed again. The emesis is nonbilious, as the hypertrophied pylorus prevents the flow of bile into the stomach (see Box 20-1). Other nonsurgical diagnoses to

Box 20-1	The importance of bilious versus nonbilious vomiting

Any vomiting in newborns should be taken seriously. Bilious emesis in a newborn should be considered a life-threatening emergency until proven otherwise and therefore should always be evaluated promptly. The presence of bile often, but not always, indicates an intestinal obstruction. In infants < 6 months of age, the most common life-threatening cause of intestinal obstruction is malrotation with midgut volvulus. Other important causes of intestinal obstruction that present in infancy include malrotation without volvulus, intestinal atresia, and Hirschsprung disease.

Box 20-2   Differential diagnosis of vomiting in an infant

Gastrointestinal
- Esophagus: stricture, web, ring, atresia
- Stomach: PS, reflux, web
- Intestine: duodenal atresia, malrotation, intussusception, incarcerated hernia, annular pancreas
- Colon: intussusception, Hirschsprung disease, imperforate anus

Infectious
- Sepsis
  - Necrotizing enterocolitis
- Meningitis
- Urinary tract infection (UTI)
- Gastroenteritis
- Pneumonia
- Otitis media
- *Bordetella pertussis*

Neurologic
- Intracranial mass lesions
  - Intracranial hemorrhage, tumor
- Cerebral edema
  - Toxins: acute lead poisoning
  - Sheering injury: shaken baby syndrome
- Hydrocephalus

Renal
- Ureteropelvic junction obstruction
- Renal tubular acidosis

Metabolic
- Inborn errors of metabolism
- Galactosemia, fructose intolerance, urea cycle defects, fatty acid oxidation disorders, amino acid and organic acid metabolism disorders

Endocrine
- Adrenal Insufficiency

Other
- Overfeeding
  - Toxic ingestion
  - Munchausen by proxy syndrome

consider in infants with nonbilious emesis include gastroenteritis, congenital adrenal hyperplasia, and inborn errors of metabolism (see Box 20-2). Physical findings will vary depending on the severity of the obstruction and the duration of symptoms. On physical examination, one can sometimes feel the hypertrophied pylorus just to the right of midline in the epigastric area. This is often referred to as the "olive." Waves of gastric peristalsis progressing from the infant's left upper abdomen to right can also be sometimes visualized just prior to emesis.

Laboratory investigation can help confirm the diagnosis if the classic triad of hypokalemia, hypochloremia, and metabolic alkalosis is found. However, this triad is often found only in the most severe cases. It results from the frequent loss of hydrogen and chloride ions from the gastric contents with a shift inward of potassium ions and outward of hydrogen ions as a compensatory effort in the setting of alkalosis. If the degree of dehydration is severe, hypernatremia and prerenal renal failure may also be found. Of note, an elevated unconjugated (indirect) bilirubin level may also be present. The exact etiology of this finding is not known, yet the indirect hyperbilirubinemia resolves quickly following surgical repair of the PS.

ETIOLOGY

The exact etiology of PS is not known. It is not believed to be congenital. Genetic factors are thought to be important, as there is an increased incidence of PS among monozygotic twins compared to dizygotic twins. It is also believed that environmental factors may interplay with genetics in the early postnatal period, such as drug exposures very early in the postnatal period. There have been reports of an association between the development of PS and the use of erythromycin in infants. It should also be noted that there is an increased rate of intestinal malrotation in patients with PS and various other associated malfor-

LITERATURE REFERENCE

 Does erythromycin increase the risk of pyloric stenosis?

Erythromycin has prominent gastrokinetic properties that have been implicated as a mechanism for promoting PS. In a retrospective study, the discharge diagnoses of 314,029 infants were reviewed. Among these infants, 0.26% were diagnosed with PS. This study showed that very early exposure to erythromycin (between 3 and 13 days of life) was associated with a nearly eightfold increased risk of PS. No increased risk of PS was seen in infants exposed to erythromycin after 13 days of life or in infants exposed to antibiotics other than erythromycin. For this reason, erythromycin is not recommended in the first 2 weeks of life [Cooper WO et al. *Arch Pediatr Adolesc Med.* 2002;156:647–650].

mations have been reported including urinary tract obstruction and esophageal atresia.

DIAGNOSIS

The diagnosis of PS is largely clinical. In an infant with progressive and forceful vomiting and an epigastric mass by examination, imaging may not be entirely necessary. However, in cases where the diagnosis is not clear from the history and examination, ultrasonography or upper gastrointestinal contrast study (UGI) can be used to help with diagnosis.

Ultrasound is the optimal diagnostic modality because it is not invasive and does not expose the infant to radiation or the risk of vomiting and aspirating contrast. The diagnosis of PS is dependent on the identification of the hypertrophic pyloric musculature and the thickness must be measured as > 4 mm with an overall pyloric diameter > 14 mm. The diagnosis can also be made if the length of the pylorus is > 26 mm. Sensitivity and specificity are both very high (> 90%) when performed by an experienced ultrasonographer.

UGI is a more invasive procedure as it requires that the infant swallow contrast and it also involves exposure to radiation; however, it can also help with the diagnosis of PS and is particularly useful when other diagnoses, such as malrotation, are being considered. The classic UGI finding for PS is an "apple core" or "string" sign, which results from the track of barium along the very thin pyloric canal. The "shoulder" sign refers to the prepyloric bulge of barium and may be visualized in the setting of PS.

TREATMENT

Think Fluid Resuscitation First

As mentioned previously, medical resuscitation takes precedence over surgical considerations. Restoring adequate hydration and electrolyte balance should be the first priority when treating these infants. Fluid boluses with isotonic crystalloid solution (e.g., NS) should be initiated. Ongoing fluid replacement should be adjusted based on clinical parameters such as skin turgor, mucous membrane moisture, heart rate, and urine output. Following appropriate bolus therapy, maintenance IV fluids should be initiated with a dextrose solution in 1/4 NS or 1/2 NS with 20 to 40 mEq/L of KCl added. Serum electrolytes and pH should be rechecked if they were abnormal at the start of therapy. Potassium replacement should be avoided unless hypokalemia is severe (e.g. K < 2 mmol/L). Potassium

LITERATURE REFERENCE

An alternative to surgery for pyloric stenosis

Although pyloromyotomy is the standard of care in the United States, studies evaluating anticholinergic drugs, such as atropine, as medical therapy for PS are ongoing in other countries and are promising as a possible alternate to surgical correction. Kawahara et al. evaluated the efficacy of atropine in patients with PS. Of the 19 enrolled infants, 17 (89%) ceased projectile vomiting after treatment with IV (median 7 days) and subsequent oral (median 44 days) atropine administration. The remaining two patients required surgery. Follow-up ultrasonography showed a significant decrease in pyloric muscle thickness after completion of the atropine treatment. No complications were reported and at 6-month follow-up all infants were reported to be thriving. While medical therapy would obviate the need for surgery, the disadvantages of this treatment option include the increased length of hospital stay (median 13 days versus 2 days with pyloromyotomy) and the necessity to continue medication administration following discharge home, often for more than 1 month. Thus far, no prospective blinded case-controlled studies have been performed and this medical therapy has not been adopted in the US [Kawahara H et al. *Arch Dis Child.* 2002;87:71–74].

replacement in infants can rapidly lead to hyperkalemia and sudden death. Hypokalemia associated with PS typically resolves spontaneously with fluid resuscitation alone.

Surgery Is the Definitive Treatment

The definitive treatment for PS is surgical correction via a procedure known as pyloromyotomy. This procedure is performed through either a very small incision at the level of the pylorus or laparoscopically through the umbilical region. The pyloric musculature is incised in a longitudinal fashion leaving only the mucosal layer intact. This alleviates the obstruction acutely, and halts the progressive thickening of the pylorus as it heals. The mortality of this procedure is < 0.5% and long-term sequelae are rare. Medical treatment for PS has been explored using anticholinergic drugs (e.g., atropine) as an alternative to surgical repair.

KEY POINTS

- Age of presentation commonly at ~1 month, range is 2 weeks to 5 months
  - 4:1 male:female ratio, white babies more commonly
  - Increased risk in first-degree family members of affected individuals
- Presents as "hungry vomiters"
  - Progressive nonbilious "projectile" emesis shortly after feeds
  - Eager to feed nearly immediately after vomiting
  - Dehydration may be severe in more protracted cases
- Classic diagnostic signs are palpable "olive" or visualized gastric peristalsis
- Classic laboratory finding is hypochloremic hypokalemic metabolic alkalosis
- Ultrasound is the diagnostic modality of choice
  - Thickened and/or elongated pylorus
- UGI may also be used for diagnosis
  - "Apple core" appearance as the barium channels through the narrowed pyloric channel
- Pyloromyotomy is the definitive treatment

CHAPTER 21

Intussusception

CASE SCENARIO

The parents of a 10-month-old girl bring her to the ED in the middle of the night because she had been having periods of irritability throughout the evening. She woke up an hour ago with a more severe episode, characterized by inconsolable crying and several bouts of nonbloody, nonbilious emesis. The entire episode lasted approximately 20 minutes and resolved on the way to the ED. She has had no diarrhea or bloody stools. She is an otherwise healthy child born at full-term. On physical examination, she is well developed, well nourished, and well appearing. She is afebrile and her pulse, respiratory rate, and blood pressure are all within normal limits for her age. Her examination is completely benign from head to toe. However, the history alarms you and you begin to consider the diagnosis of intussusception.

1. Which of the following is not a classic feature of intussusception?
   a. Female gender
   b. Age 10 months
   c. Colicky pain
   d. Nonbilious emesis

Intussusception can happen in any gender; however, it occurs in boys at least twice as often as girls. The most common age of presentation is from 6 months to 2 years. The pain is often intermittent in nature and it is not uncommon for a patient to be completely well appearing on initial examination early in the course of the illness. Thus, early diagnosis of intussusception often requires a high clinical suspicion from history and epidemiologic factors alone. Emesis is often present. Initially it is nonbilious, yet as the obstruction progresses and becomes complete, the emesis may become bilious.

2. Which of the following can be seen in intussusception?
   a. Mass in the right upper quadrant
   b. Dance's sign
   c. High-pitched bowel sounds
   d. Absent bowel sounds
   e. All of the above

All of the above findings can be found in the setting of intussusception. The mass in the right upper quadrant is sometimes referred to as a "sausage" and represents the portion of intestine that has in effect telescoped into the downstream portion of bowel, forming a palpable mass. When this occurs at the ileocolic junction, which is the most common site of intussusception, the portion of bowel that usually rests in the right lower quadrant, referred to as the *intussusceptum*, is displaced into the receiving portion of bowel, the *intussuscipiens*, in the right upper quadrant, thus leaving the right lower quadrant relatively empty. The absence of bowel contents on abdominal x-ray in the right lower quadrant is referred to as *Dance's sign*. In the early phases of intussusception, high-pitched bowel sounds representing the formation of an obstruction may be present. Once the obstruction is complete, and if the bowel has become damaged, peristalsis will halt and bowel sounds will decrease; they may be absent altogether.

While you are still in the room with this patient, she suddenly draws her legs up to her abdomen and begins to cry. You again examine her abdomen and this time you are able to appreciate a mass in the right upper quadrant, suggestive of intussusception.

3. What should be your next step in this patient's management?
   a. Obtain a surgical consult
   b. Place an IV and initiate a 20 cc/kg NS bolus
   c. Perform an abdominal ultrasound
   d. Perform a contrast enema

All of the above will likely take place as the care of this patient evolves. However, given the high clinical suspicion for intussusception in this case, placement of an IV and administration of a fluid bolus should take place first before any diagnostic or therapeutic procedures. Even though our patient does not appear dehydrated, she is at risk for significant fluid loss through her likely edematous bowel. Abdominal ultrasound is almost always diagnostic and a contrast enema (air, barium, or water-soluble contrast) can be both diagnostic and therapeutic. Contrast enemas are performed by a radiologist, however, only in the presence of a surgeon in case of complications that would require surgical intervention. Surgery is often not necessary for reduction of the intussusception, which most often can be reduced with a contrast enema (80 to 90% success rate). The risks include intestinal perforation and incomplete reduction, but these complications are rare.

Your patient is diagnosed with an ileocolic intussusception by air enema, and it is subsequently reduced by air enema successfully without any complications. Her parents inquire about the chances that this will happen again.

4. What is the risk of recurrence?
   a. 1%
   b. 10%
   c. 25%
   d. 50%

In patients with successful enema reduction, the recurrence risk is about 10%. This risk is greatest within the first 24 hours following reduction; therefore, patients are hospitalized for observation during this period.

Answers: 1-a, 2-e, 3-b, 4-b

DEFINITION

Intussusception is defined as a segment of bowel sliding, or telescoping, forward through a segment of bowel just distal to it. This can occur anywhere along the alimentary tract, yet it occurs most often at the ileocolic junction where the ileum invaginates into the colon, accounting for more than 75% of cases (see Figure 21-1). The proximal telescoping portion is often referred to as the intussusceptum and the distal receiving portion as the intussuscipiens. Intussusception is the most common cause of intestinal obstruction in children. Its incidence is estimated at 1 to 4 in 1,000 live births. It is very rare in neonates and typically occurs between the ages of 6 months and 6 years with approximately 60% of cases occurring in patients < 1 year and 80% of all cases occurring by 2 years of age. Boys are affected at least twice as often as girls with male:female ratios ranging between 2:1 and 6:1. Some cases resolve spontaneously but often recur.

If unrecognized and left untreated intussusception will progress to local bowel ischemia, perforation, and death.

CLINICAL PRESENTATION

Intussusception most commonly presents as intermittent and relatively frequent episodes of crampy abdominal pain in a previously healthy child. Initially children are quite well appearing in between episodes, often becoming more lethargic as the obstruction worsens. Intussusception is typically accompanied in the early stages by nonbilious emesis, which transitions to bilious emesis as the obstruction becomes more complete.

Lower gastrointestinal (GI) bleeding is the hallmark of intussusception. Stools are hemoccult positive in > 80% of cases. Roughly half of patients will pass stools with dark blood clots and mucous, commonly through peristalsis to invaginate itself into the distal fixed portion. Some examples of lead-points include Meckel's diverticulum, intestinal polyps and neoplasms, the appendix, and foreign bodies. Patients with Henoch-Schonlein purpura and hemophilia have an increased incidence of intussusception, believed secondary to submucosal hemorrhage acting as a mechanical lead-point.

Hypertrophic Peyer's patches, or intestinal lymph nodes, are thought to be a common lead-point. This can be in response to a viral gastroenteritis or any other abdominal process that causes reactive lymph nodes. In fact, intussusception has a seasonal variation with its prevalence being higher during the time of year that viral gastroenteritis is prevalent. Intussusception can also occur in the post operative period in patients who have undergone abdominal surgery. However, despite many known mechanical lead-points, > 80% of pediatric cases do not have an identifiable pathologic lead-point, although the identification of lead-points increases proportionately with age.

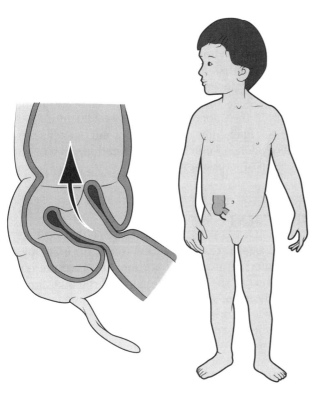

FIGURE 21-1 Intussusception—Illustration of the anatomy of the ileocecal junction where intussusception has occurred; (left) a portion of the ileum has been pushed into the lumen of the adjoining cecum; (right) child is shown standing with location of ileocecal junction indicated. (*From LifeART image copyright © 2005 Lippincott Williams & Wilkins. All rights reserved.*)

referred to as the classic "currant jelly" stool. This develops later in the course as bowel ischemia develops with venous congestion, mucosal sloughing, and subsequent bleeding. Eventually, if not recognized, intussusception will lead to bowel infarction and death.

The classic physical examination findings include a sausage-like mass representing the intussusception in the right upper quadrant, often oriented along the cephalocaudad axis. This finding may or may not be accompanied by a relative absence of bowel in the right lower quadrant on abdominal x-ray, referred to as Dance's sign. Otherwise the physical examination varies depending on the degree of obstruction or bowel ischemia.

ETIOLOGY

The cause of intussusception in most cases is not identified. Some cases are attributed to a mechanical lead-point, meaning a structure adjacent to or attached to the bowel lumen fixing it in place. A lead-point can allow a more mobile proximal segment of bowel

DIAGNOSIS

An air or contrast enema is the test of choice in cases where intussusception is suspected (i.e., intermittent abdominal pain or irritability, hemoccult positive or bloody stools). The bowel is insufflated with air or contrast (barium or water soluble) while fluoroscopy is being performed (i.e., real-time x-ray). The classic finding is described as the "meniscus" sign, which is produced by the rounded leading edge of the intussusceptum protruding into the more distal air or contrast filled bowel. The advantage to air or contrast enema is that this maneuver will often reduce the intussusception; therefore, this modality acts as treatment in addition to its diagnostic capability.

Ultrasound is often preferred as the first test because it is less invasive, especially in cases where the clinical suspicion is not as high. Ultrasound has a 98% sensitivity for the diagnosis of intussusception. Classic ultrasound findings include a tubular mass in longitudinal views, sometimes referred to as a "pseudokidney," and a doughnut or target appearance in transverse images. Doppler ultrasound can also give information regarding blood flow and bowel wall ischemia. Saline enema under ultrasound surveillance is becoming increasingly popular as it avoids radiation exposure, although it is not yet regarded as standard of care.

Plain abdominal radiographs can also be useful in the diagnosis of intussusception. They can be suggestive of the diagnosis when a right upper quadrant mass is present, often obscuring the lower liver margin. Other signs suggestive of intussusception, although

LITERATURE REFERENCE

Should ultrasound be used as a screening tool in suspected cases of intussusception?

Henrickson et al. looked at children with suspected intussusception to determine the usefulness of ultrasound as a screening tool prior to fluoroscopy with enemas in an effort to reduce unnecessary radiation exposure in children. They found that prior to the introduction of ultrasound screening, only 20% of children who underwent fluoroscopic enema had intussusception and thus the majority was needlessly exposed to radiation and the risk of perforation via an enema. Screening ultrasound showed a negative predictive value of 100% (i.e., no false-positives leading to subsequent fluoroscopy), and the subsequent rate of positive enema studies increased from 20% to nearly 60%. Although the sample size is on the low side (n=40), this study suggests that screening ultrasound is a useful tool to limit unnecessary exposure to radiation and discomfort in children with suspected intussusception **[Henrickson et al. *Pediatr Radiol*. 2003;33(3):190–193].**

LITERATURE REFERENCE

Can ultrasound diagnose and treat intussusception?

Gonzalez-Spinola et al. evaluated the therapeutic value of ultrasound-guided saline enema for the reduction of intussusception in nearly 200 patients in Spain. They achieved a success rate as high as 88% with hydrostatic saline reduction using ultrasound guidance. In 15% of cases a second attempt 30 minutes after the initial attempt was required to achieve reduction. There were no associated perforations. These success rates are comparable to conventional enema with fluoroscopy and is evidence supporting ultrasound-guided reduction **[Gonzalez-Spinola J et al. *J Pediatr Surg*. 1999; 34(6):1016–1020].**

not entirely specific, include reduced amount of air in the small intestine, a gasless abdomen, or other signs suggestive of a bowel obstruction, including air fluid levels. Visualization of a normal cecum filled with either air or feces points away from intussusception. This assumes of course that intussusception only occurs at the ileocolic junction, which is not always the case. Plain films can also be useful to exclude free air as evidence for intestinal perforation, a major complication of intussusception.

TREATMENT

The success rate of reduction under fluoroscopy or ultrasound is directly proportional to the duration of symptoms. If the procedure is performed within the first 48 hours of symptoms, the success rate is approximately 80% to 90%. The success rate is only 50% in cases where symptoms have persisted > 48 hours. The rate of bowel perforation with the use of barium or saline enemas is roughly 0.5% to 2.5%. The perforation rate with air reduction is less, ranging from 0.1% to 0.2%.

Enema reduction is contraindicated if signs of frank bowel ischemia or perforation already exist, including peritonitis or shock, or radiographic evidence of free intraperitoneal air or pneumatosis intestinalis (i.e., air in the bowel wall indicative of bowel wall infarction). In these cases, surgical exploration is necessary to mechanically reduce the intussusception and assess the need for bowel resection (see Box 21-1). Surgical reduction is also recommended for recurrent

---

BOX 21-1   Surgical reduction of intussusception

Surgical reduction is necessary when conventional enema reduction fails, or when it is contraindicated due to either the presence of peritoneal signs with suspected bowel perforation, or a history of multiple recurrent episodes. Typically, a transverse incision is made in the right side of the abdomen and the intussusceptum is located through this incision. Reduction is achieved by manually squeezing the mass from the distal to proximal portion in a retrograde fashion until the bowel is completely reduced. Bowel integrity is next assessed and warm packs may be placed on any involved segment that has questionable viability to facilitate blood flow. In cases where the intussusception can not be reduced in this fashion, or if a lead-point of necrotic bowel is identified, a bowel resection is necessary, typically an ileocolectomy with primary reanastomosis. The recurrence rate with surgical reduction is estimated to be 3%, and <1% with surgical resection.

intussusception (particularly after the third occurrence), for cases of a known pathologic lead-point, and for cases where enema reduction is unsuccessful.

Following enema reduction the recurrence rate of intussusception is approximately 10%. Surgical reductions are associated with a lower incidence of recurrence, approximately 3%. When surgery involves bowel resection due to the presence of necrotic bowel or a lead-point, the recurrence rate is near zero.

KEY POINTS

- Intussusception is the most common cause of intestinal obstruction in children
  - Rare in neonates
  - Eighty percent of cases occur between 6 months and 2 years of life
  - Boys affected at least twice as often as girls
- Lead-points are rare in children; however, their incidence increases with age
- Ileocolic region is the most common site of occurrence
- Index of suspicion must be high based on history
  - Intermittent colic and irritability followed by periods of normal behavior
- Classic examination findings include palpation of a tubular mass ("sausage") in right upper quadrant and GI bleeding
  - Hemoccult positive stools in 80%
  - "Currant jelly" stool is classic yet occurs in < 50%
- Air and contrast enemas under fluoroscopy have been the standard
  - Risk of perforation and require radiation
  - Provides therapy as well as diagnostics
- Ultrasound is less invasive and has a high sensitivity
- Also has the potential to identify lead-points if present
- Abdominal plain films are not sensitive
- Most intussusceptions are successfully reduced by air or contrast enema
- Surgical reduction is required in several circumstances
  - Repeated unsuccessful attempts at enema reduction
  - The presence of an identifiable lead-point requiring resection
  - Suspicion for perforation or bowel necrosis

Practice Cases

CASE 1

A 13-year-old girl is brought to the ED by her parents for fever. The patient's history is significant for acute lymphoblastic leukemia (ALL) diagnosed 4 months ago. She has been receiving chemotherapy every few weeks as an inpatient in the hospital; her last admission was 3 weeks ago. Her parents are unsure what chemotherapy she received. At home, she is seen by a visiting nurse who draws blood for complete blood count (CBC) twice a week from her Broviac catheter and reports them to her oncologist. Her counts were normal 3 days ago according to her parents. She has not recently required any transfusions of platelets or red blood cells (RBC), but has received them in the past. She was acting normally yesterday evening and was playing with her younger sisters without any problems. Her 8-year-old sister has had a runny nose and cough but no fever over the past few days. This morning she slept later than usual and her parents checked her temperature, which was 103.2°F orally. Review of systems is negative for cough, headache, abdominal pain, nausea, vomiting, diarrhea, or rash. They called their oncologist who sent her to the ED immediately for evaluation.

1. What is the most concerning aspect of her initial history?
   a. Fever to 103°F
   b. History of ALL with recent chemotherapy
   c. History of blood transfusions
   d. Sister with rhinorrhea and cough

In this patient presenting with fever, the most concerning aspect is her history of ALL, which suggest she is in an immunocompromised state. Her history of chemotherapy has likely affected her immune system and made her susceptible to infection. Height of fever does have a significant correlation with risk of bacterial illness, especially in children under 36 months. Older children may also have high fever with viruses, and they are not as susceptible to serious bacterial infection (SBI) as young children. However, ALL makes her susceptible to bacterial illness, and a fever in this setting must be taken seriously. Blood and platelet transfusions are common in children undergoing chemotherapy. They may cause fever during infusion, but that is not the case here. They carry a small risk of infection, but are not likely contributing to this acute presentation. Her sister with cough and runny nose suggest a viral illness that may be the cause of her fever; this deserves further investigation.

The patient's vital signs reveal a temperature of 102.6°F, heart rate (HR) of 130 beats per minute (bpm), blood pressure of 105/49 mm Hg, respiratory rate of 20, and pulse oximetry of 98%. Her physical examination reveals a young girl with thinning alopecia who is otherwise well appearing. She has normal tympanic membranes, no nasal discharge and a normal-appearing pharynx. Her lungs are clear and heart is tachycardic with a regular rate. Her abdomen is soft and nontender. Extremities are warm with a capillary refill less than 2 seconds. Labs are drawn off her indwelling catheter, including a CBC with differential, blood culture, and electrolytes. A nasal swab is sent for influenza.

2. While awaiting her laboratory results, the most important priority is
   a. Acetaminophen by mouth
   b. Oral hydration
   c. Intravenous (IV) broad-spectrum antibiotics
   d. Contacting the oncologist regarding type of chemotherapeutic agents

In an immunocompromised patient with fever, the most appropriate therapy is IV antibiotics. She is at risk for infection with both gram-positive and gram-negative organisms and antibiotics should cover against both. It is somewhat reassuring that her recent CBC was normal, but this cannot exclude a serious infection in an immunocompromised patient. Acetaminophen (Tylenol) should be given to lower her temperature for patient comfort but is not as important as early antibiotic administration. Additionally, fluids may be appropriate as she is tachycardic; this may be secondary to dehydration and fever. The primary oncologist should also be contacted early in order to obtain as much information as possible regarding the patient's recent management.

You consult her oncologist who confirms that her last CBC did not reveal neutropenia. The decision is made to administer IV cefepime, as it has broad coverage against gram-positive and gram-negative organisms. You also administer Tylenol 500 mg orally and a 500 cc fluid bolus. Her CBC reveals a normal white blood cell (WBC) count and differential, hematocrit of 28, and platelets of 190. You are reassured that she is not neutropenic. IV cefepime has been administered. During re examination, you note that her blood pressure has fallen to 90/40, and her HR continues at 130 bpm. She looks a bit pale but her capillary refill remains less than 2 seconds. She feels better after the fluid bolus and Tylenol.

3. What is the appropriate intervention?
    a. Administer isotonic saline bolus 20 cc/kg (1 liter)
    b. Start a dopamine infusion through her central line
    c. Start a norepinephrine infusion
    d. Perform endotracheal intubation

The patient has dropped her blood pressure below age-specific criteria for hypotension using the formula $70 + (age \times 2)$ for systolic blood pressure. The immediate concern is septic shock. In this case, a normal capillary refill suggests warm shock secondary to peripheral vasodilatation. An immediate fluid bolus over 20 minutes should be given. Dopamine and norepinephrine are important vasopressors that are used in persistent fluid-resistant shock, but aggressive fluid resuscitation should be attempted first. The patient is alert, talkative, and has no evidence of a deteriorating airway; intubation is not necessary.

After 20 minutes, the patient is still alert, but she looks and feels ill. Her HR is 120 bpm but her blood pressure is now 85/35 mm Hg. Her distal pulses are brisk with adequate capillary refill. An additional 20 cc/kg bolus is given over 20 minutes. Her HR is rechecked at 110 bpm and her blood pressure has improved to 95/40 mm Hg. Lungs are clear bilaterally. Given her low blood pressure likely secondary to sepsis, you decide to add vancomycin to expand gram-positive coverage and gentamicin to double-cover for gram-negative organisms. An hour later, her rate has again risen to 130 bpm and blood pressure fallen to 83/38 mm Hg.

The patient is given a third bolus, but despite this, her blood pressure falls to 85/42 mm Hg. She vomits some ginger ale that you gave her.

4. What is the next step in management?
    a. Additional fluid boluses
    b. Endotracheal intubation to maximize oxygen delivery
    c. Start a dopamine infusion and admit to the ICU
    d. Provide an antiemetic

The patient has received three fluid boluses with transient effects and now is again hypotensive. Starting a vasopressor in addition to more fluid would now be appropriate. Patients with sepsis are significantly volume depleted and should receive aggressive fluid resuscitation. However, sepsis is mediated through circulating endotoxins that result in hypotension by several mechanisms. One is by third-spacing of fluids from intravascular to extravascular spaces, resulting in intravascular volume depletion. Hypotension is also a result of decreased peripheral vascular tone, resulting in vasodilation, and impaired cardiac output. For the last two reasons, if aggressive fluid resuscitation alone does not improve tissue perfusion, a vasopressor must be added. The patient is transported to the ICU and supported with fluids and a dopamine infusion. Twelve hours later, her blood culture grows gram-positive cocci in clusters. Line sepsis is suspected and she is continued on antibiotics; the central line is immediately removed. Dopamine is slowly weaned off and her condition continues to improve. *Staphylococcus aureus* sensitive to vancomycin grows from blood culture. Catheter tip culture also grows *S. aureus*.

Answers: 1-b, 2-c, 3-a, 4-c

CASE 2

A 4-week-old female infant presents to the ED for vomiting. She is the product of a full-term vaginal delivery with no complications at birth. She went home from the nursery after 2 days. She has been breast-feeding well and gaining weight appropriately. Physical examinations were normal at 2 and 4 weeks of age. Yesterday evening she began vomiting small amounts after breast-feeding. The vomiting has increased in frequency and is now a bright yellow color. Some of the episodes of vomiting were very forceful and went across the room. Mom has not thought she felt warm so did not check a temperature. There are no other children at home and no one else is sick. There has been no cough, runny nose, diarrhea, or rash.

5. What is the most likely cause of projectile vomiting at this age?
    a. Pyloric stenosis (PS)
    b. Volvulus
    c. Malrotation
    d. Duodenal atresia
    e. Sepsis

PS commonly presents at this age-group with projectile vomiting. Onset is usually a gradual increase in frequency of vomiting and this patient's history is very suspicious for PS. Volvulus and a malrotation leading to volvulus are important causes of acute bilious vomiting in this age range and should also be considered. Duodenal atresia usually presents in the first few hours of life and would not present like this patient. Sepsis should always be entertained in a vomiting neonate and temperature should be checked.

On physical examination, the patient is irritable and crying. Temperature is 98.6°F, HR 160 bpm, blood pressure 78/50 mm Hg, respiratory rate 40, and pulse oximetry 98%. Anterior fontanelle is open and flat. Lungs are clear and heart is regular rate and rhythm. Abdomen is slightly distended with diminished bowel sounds and is difficult to palpate secondary to crying. She has normal genitourinary examination. You inform mom not to give her any more breast milk. An abdominal ultrasound is ordered. Ultrasound reveals a thickness of 3 mm and a length of 10 mm for the pylorus which is not consistent with PS. A pediatric surgery consult is obtained and they suggest additional testing including laboratory tests and an upper gastrointestinal (UGI) contrast study.

6. What are the common electrolytes abnormalities found in PS?
    a. Hyperchloremic, hyperkalemic metabolic acidosis
    b. Hyperchloremic, hypokalemic metabolic acidosis
    c. Hypochloremic, hyperkalemic metabolic alkalosis
    d. Hypochloremic, hypokalemic metabolic alkalosis

Patients with PS have vomiting of their stomach secretions and subsequent loss of electrolytes. This includes the loss of hydrogen ions, leading to an alkalosis. Additionally, both chloride and potassium are lost. Thus, the classic laboratory findings are a hypochloremic, hypokalemic metabolic alkalosis.

Labs are drawn and an IV is placed. During the procedure, the patient has additional vomiting which you note to be bright green. You inform pediatric surgery and order an emergent UGI.

7. Now that PS is less likely, what diagnosis is now of concern and the reason for obtaining an UGI?
    a. Appendicitis
    b. Duodenal atresia
    c. Volvulus
    d. Intussusception
    e. Necrotizing enterocolitis (NEC)

Bilious vomiting in a neonate is a surgical emergency. The most important diagnosis to think of is malrotation with midgut volvulus because delay in surgical correction can lead to extensive gut necrosis. While the other problems also require prompt diagnosis and treatment, they are usually diagnosed by other means. The diagnosis of duodenal atresia is typically made by plain radiography with the "double-bubble sign." NEC is diagnosed by plain radiographs as well. Intussusception can be diagnosed by a number of methods including plain radiographs and ultrasound; however, barium enema remains the gold standard. Appendicitis can also be confirmed through computed tomography (CT) imaging, with the best method involving rectal contrast.

The patient has an UGI performed. There is no evidence of a "string sign" that would suggest PS. Contrast does not cross the midline and remains on the patient's right side. Additionally there is a corkscrew appearance of the contrast which suddenly stops in a "beak" appearance. The radiologist informs you this is highly suspicious for a malrotation with midgut volvulus. Pediatric surgery is informed and prepares the OR. The patient continues to have small amounts of bilious emesis. Her vitals remain stable except for tachycardia for which you initiate IV fluids. You are concerned about aspiration, given the degree of vomiting.

8. What is the easiest intervention to help decrease the patient's risk of aspiration before surgery?
    a. Intubation
    b. Nasogastric (NG) tube
    c. Raise head of the bed
    d. Make patient non per os (NPO)

The patient is already NPO in preparation for surgery, but it does not diminish the production of gastric secretions. Intubation will be performed in the OR and does not necessarily need to be urgently performed in the ED. Placing an NG tube will help suction gastric secretions and is a quick and easy intervention. The length of the NG tube can be estimated from the distance between the patient's nose to angle of the mandible to the xiphoid process of the sternum and inserted into the patient's nose to that depth. Suction should obtain gastric secretions. Placement can also be confirmed by injecting 3 cc of air into the tubing and listening at the stomach with a stethoscope for a gush of air. Raising the head of the bed may be appropriate for patients with reflux but is not appropriate in this situation.

The patient is brought to the OR and is intubated. A malrotation with volvulus is confirmed. The intestines are easily reduced and there is no evidence of necrosis. A Ladd procedure is performed and the patient is brought to the recovery room without incident. The patient is observed in the hospital and resumed on oral breast-feeding. After 3 days, the patient is tolerating fluids and is released from the hospital.

Answers: 5-a, 6-d, 7-c, 8-b

CASE 3

A 4-month-old child arrives in the ED by ambulance after having reportedly fallen from her high chair. Her parents arrive shortly thereafter and report that she lost consciousness for approximately 1 minute at the scene after appearing to land on her shoulder and head. They remark that she was fussing and squirming and that her movement caused the high chair to fall over, while she remained belted inside. After a period of unresponsiveness, she then awoke and was moving all extremities without difficulty, clinging to her mother while crying. They deny any seizure activity. Paramedics report that she remained irritable en route to the hospital but that she continued to have normal vital signs. In the ED, she is placed on a monitor, given supplemental O_2, and IV access is obtained. She continues to be alert and appropriate, but very fussy. Her examination is significant for an impressive hematoma over her right parietal region and you palpate an irregularity in her skull in the same region. She has no gross neurologic abnormalities, but a complete examination is limited by her age and lack of cooperation, although you note that her anterior fontanelle feels remarkably full.

9. What is the next appropriate step in her management?
    a. Observe for 4 hours in the ED
    b. Obtain an IV contrast head CT
    c. Obtain a head CT without IV contrast
    d. Obtain a head MRI

This patient is at high risk of suffering from intracranial injury (ICI) given her young age, loss of consciousness for possibly longer than 1 minute, and physical examination findings that are suspicious for a skull fracture, in addition to her continued irritability. Patients at high risk for ICI require head imaging and noncontrast head CT is the best testing modality to look for acute intracranial bleeds.

While waiting for her head CT, she develops several forceful bouts of nonbloody emesis and continues to be extremely irritable. Ten minutes later the nurse notifies you that she has started to seize. The parents report that it started with left sided "twitching" movements and that she had become unresponsive just prior to onset of the "jerking" motions. You observe generalized tonic-clonic movements associated with perioral cyanosis. You immediately administer supplemental oxygen.

10. What is your next step in her management?
    a. Administer lorazepam 0.1 mg/kg IV
    b. Administer diazepam 0.5 mg/kg per rectum (PR)
    c. Administer phenobarbital and intubate
    d. Administer pentobarbital and intubate

The first step in seizure management involves the administration of a benzodiazepine, favoring lorazepam if IV access is immediately available, as it is in this case scenario, for any child who seizes for greater than 5 minutes or who has evidence of airway compromise. In addition, when head injury is suspected, seizures should be treated aggressively as they further increase cerebral blood flow and thereby raise intracranial pressure (ICP) even further. Barbiturates are typically considered third-line therapy behind benzodiazepines and phenytoin. Although when seizures occur in a setting where there is a high risk of increased ICP, barbiturates are often used earlier rather than later, and pentobarbital is preferred due to its ability to lower ICP.

You administer lorazepam 0.1 mg/kg IV. She continues to seize and within 2 minutes, you note that her pulse is falling and her respirations are becoming irregular.

11. What is your next step?
    a. Rapid sequence intubation
    b. Administer a second dose of Ativan (lorazepam)
    c. Administer mannitol
    d. Call for stat neurosurgery consult

Any patient with bradycardia, hypertension, and irregular respirations (Cushing's triad) is suffering from increased ICP and at severe risk for cerebral herniation. Young infants are at less of a risk for this given their open fontanelles, but in the setting of severe bleeds, they too can herniate and die. As always, protecting the patient's airway must be your first priority, but in this case you also need to do everything possible to reduce her ICP immediately until more definitive neurosurgical intervention can take place. You immediately intubate using etomidate and Succinylcholine and hyperventilate, which results in hypocarbia and transiently decreases ICP. Her seizures stop following a pentobarbital bolus and you place her on a pentobarbital drip. You also administer mannitol 0.5 g/kg IV and accompany her to the CT scanner.

12. What findings do you suspect account for her acute decompensation?
    a. Subdural hematoma
    b. Epidural hematoma
    c. Diffuse axonal injury
    d. Parietal skull fracture
    e. Midline shift

The patient's history is most suspicious for an epidural hematoma, "the walk, talk, and die" type of intracranial bleed. These bleeds commonly follow a brief loss of consciousness, then a lucid interval subsequently, and followed by acute decompensation as the arterial hematoma expands. Her clinical picture is highly suspicious for cerebral herniation, and midline shift, as a result of the expanding hematoma. Epidural hemorrhage is usually associated with a skull fracture and tearing of the middle meningeal artery.

As predicted, the head CT shows a large right parietal epidural bleed with midline shift and a depressed parietal skull fracture. She returns to the ED from radiology and is evaluated by pediatric neurosurgery who take her emergently to the OR for drainage of the bleed and placement of a temporary externalized ventricular drain and ICP monitor.

Despite her aggressive clinical management, the patient decompensates and dies later the same evening in the ICU. Autopsy reveals other associated findings.

13. Which of the following might you expect?
    a. Multiple posterior rib fractures
    b. Retinal hemorrhages
    c. Femur fracture
    d. Diffuse axonal injury
    e. All of the above

Never miss a case of nonaccidental trauma! Always suspect foul play when a story does not make sense or does not fit the injury, or when you receive conflicting stories from different caregivers, or even when you just get the sense that something is off. It is always worth further inquisition and investigation by multiple medical caregivers in the emergency setting including social workers and members of the child protection team, as well as consultation with the patient's primary care physician (PCP) to try to gather as much information as possible regarding the safety of the child. Remember, you are responsible for the patient's safety, and should also be thinking of the safety of any other children who may be in the household.

In this case, the patient was a victim of nonaccidental trauma and had been shaken repeatedly when she would not stop crying. When she cried more, her mother threw her down in frustration onto the bed, from which she fell to the hardwood floor, landing on her head. Hopefully you suspected this from the start of this case scenario, as 3-month-old children should not even be in high chairs and certainly are not capable of generating the force required to flip themselves over. The mechanism of injury is not age-appropriate and therefore should have raised suspicion early on in the management of this case.

Answers: 9-c, 10-a, 11-a, 12-b, 13-e

CASE 4

A 3-year-old boy with a prior history of asthma is referred to your ED by his PCP for persistent respiratory distress in the setting of frequent nebulizer treatments. His mother reports that he has been having a runny nose and cough with low-grade fevers for 2 days. Over the course of the night prior to presentation, his cough worsened and he developed increased work of breathing that was only temporarily relieved by albuterol nebulizer treatments. His mother reports giving treatments initially every 4 hours, but most recently she had been administering nebulizer therapy every 2 hours. On presentation to the ED, his temperature is 100.4°F orally, HR 120, respiratory rate 42, blood pressure 95/60, and oxygen saturation 94% on room air (RA). On physical examination, he is in nontoxic but in moderate respiratory distress with supracostal and subcostal retractions. Air exchange is moderate and symmetric with diffuse wheezing but without evidence for focal consolidation. His cardiac examination does not reveal any murmur and the remainder of his examination is normal except for some clear rhinorrhea.

14. What is your first step in his management?
    a. Administer albuterol nebulizer 2.5 mg × 1
    b. Administer albuterol nebulizer 2.5 mg × 3 in rapid succession
    c. Administer albuterol 2.5 mg neb with Atrovent (ipratropium bromide) 500-mcg neb × 1
    d. Administer albuterol 2.5 mg neb with Atrovent 500 mcg × 3

Atrovent has been shown to reduce admissions from the ED when given in combination with albuterol (Combivent). Initial studies showed that one administration of Combivent followed by two straight albuterol nebs reduced admission rates. A more recent follow-up study suggests that the efficacy may be increased when all three "stacked" treatments are albuterol combined with Atrovent.

While the patient is receiving his stacked treatments, you obtain a more detailed history from his mother. She reports that he uses his albuterol at least twice daily, even when he is well. During upper respiratory illnesses, he typically develops a worsening cough and respiratory distress. He has had two hospitalizations as an infant for respiratory distress, requiring supplemental oxygen and she recalls at least two prior courses of steroids. She reports that he once developed a severe rash while taking amoxicillin.

15. What is the next best step in his management?
    a. Obtain a chest x-ray
    b. Administer prednisone 2 mg/kg PO
    c. Administer Solu-Medrol (methyl-prednisolone sodium succinate) 2 mg/kg IV
    d. Administer amoxicillin 80 mg/kg/day in three doses

Early administration of steroids is imperative in the management of known asthmatics who present in significant respiratory distress. This patient is in moderate distress and does not appear to be declining further. He is an appropriate candidate for oral steroids. In patients who are in severe distress and incapable of swallowing medication, or whom you are concerned that you may need to intubate and therefore you want to keep NPO, then IV steroid administration is appropriate. A chest x-ray is indicated in anybody who does not carry a known history of asthma and wheezing. It is also indicated in any patient with asymmetric findings on lung examination or in anyone with concern for pneumonia or foreign body aspiration by history alone. Antibiotics should not be administered unless a presumed bacterial infection (e.g., infiltrate on chest x-ray, otitis media) is identified. This patient does not have any focal findings on his examination suggestive of such and therefore antibiotics would not be an appropriate choice of therapy at this point in his care.

He receives steroids and then finishes the three nebulizer treatments. He responds very well with increased oxygen saturations on room air to 98% and a decreased respiratory rate to 24. He continues to have scattered wheezes on examination but has excellent aeration throughout. His mother is requesting to take him home. You observe him in the ED for a total of 3 hours and he remains very active and in no acute distress. You discharge him home on a 5-day course of prednisone 2 mg/kg and albuterol 2.5 mg nebulized q4h and arrange follow-up with his PCP on the following day.

Three days later, he returns to the ED. His mother never took him for his follow-up evaluation because he continued to do well with nebulizer treatments every 4 hours and prednisone, although she reports that today he vomited immediately following the prednisone. Today, he acutely worsened in the setting of a new fever to 104.2°F orally. His fever is confirmed in the ED and his HR is elevated at 145, as is his respiratory rate at 62. He is hypoxic with a room air saturation of 88%. His lung examination reveals suprasternal, intercostal, and subcostal retractions with diffuse wheezes and decreased aeration, particularly in the right base.

16. What is your first management step?
    a. Albuterol/Atrovent nebulizer treatment
    b. Obtain a chest x-ray
    c. Apply supplemental oxygen
    d. Place an IV for Solu-Medrol administration

Evaluation of the airway, breathing, and circulation (ABCs) always takes precedence. This patient is in moderate to severe respiratory distress and is hypoxic. He needs oxygen before anything else. A Combivent nebulizer treatment should be administered as soon as possible. His history of worsening fever and respiratory distress and his asymmetric lung examination are suspicious for the development of a focal process, such as pneumonia. Therefore, a chest x-ray is reasonable; however, this should not be performed until his respiratory status improves. IV Solu-Medrol is no more efficacious than oral prednisone and therefore Solu-Medrol need not be administered in place of prednisone unless he is at a risk for vomiting.

After receiving nebulizer treatments, his distress improves significantly, but he remains mildly hypoxic, at 93% on 2L O_2 by nasal canula. He travels to radiology with an oxygen tank. Chest x-ray reveals an infiltrate in his right middle lobe, as you had suspected. You start an IV, administer a 20 cc/kg fluid bolus and ceftriaxone 50 mg/kg. Five minutes after the medication is hung, the nurse calls you because he has developed hives. While you are in the room evaluating him, you note increasing respiratory distress and he begins to complain that his tongue feels "funny."

17. What is your first step?
    a. Administer diphenhydramine 1 mg/kg IV
    b. Administer epinephrine (1:1,000) 0.01 mg/kg intramuscularly (IM)
    c. Administer epinephrine 0.01 mg/kg (1:10,000) IV
    d. Discontinue the ceftriaxone infusion immediately

You suspect an allergic reaction and immediately discontinue the ceftriaxone. You then increase his supplemental oxygen and obtain a complete set of vital signs. The nurse simultaneously administers epinephrine (1:1,000) 0.01 mg/kg IM. One minute following the administration of epinephrine, his vital signs are a pulse of 170, respiratory rate 42, blood pressure 78/50, and oxygen saturation 100% on 10 L O_2 face mask. The patient appears sleepy but remains arousable.

18. What is your next step?
    a. Administer another dose of IM epinephrine at 0.01 mg/kg
    b. Administer epinephrine IV
    c. Administer a 20 cc/kg NS bolus
    d. Start dopamine 5 mcg/kg/min IV

While this patient's blood pressure is still within "normal" range for his age, it has fallen significantly since his admission to the ED and he is beginning to show signs of decreased cerebral perfusion with his declining mental status. His oxygen saturation remains 100% on supplemental oxygen, and thus you suspect his symptoms are due to decreased cerebral perfusion rather than hypoxia. Hypotension here is a result of dehydration from tachypnea and vasodilation associated with anaphylaxis. Therefore, an additional NS bolus is indicated followed by further epinephrine if hypoperfusion persists.

19. What additional treatments are indicated at this point in time?
     a. Diphenhydramine 1 mg/kg IV
     b. Ranitidine 1 mg/kg IV
     c. Solu-Medrol 2 mg/kg IV
     d. All of the above

While epinephrine is first-line therapy in anaphylaxis, all of the above medications are considered adjunctive therapy and should be administered as soon as possible in patients with anaphylactic shock. Steroids will play an important role, particularly in our patient with his history of asthma and intercurrent flair of pneumonia.

Eight minutes following the first dose of epinephrine, the patient has improved significantly. His blood pressure is up to 90/60 and his oxygen saturation remains stable on 2 L of supplemental oxygen. You keep him in the ED for observation for several hours and then transfer him to the floor for further observation and management of his pneumonia and asthma. You conclude that he had a type 1 hypersensitivity reaction to ceftriaxone.

Answers: 14-d, 15-b, 16-c, 17-d, 18-c, 19-d

CASE 5

A 9-day-old boy born full term without pregnancy or delivery complications is brought into the ED by his mother because she is concerned that he has a cough and cold and that he is not eating well. She reports that he was initially a vigorous feeder but over the past 24 hours she feels that he has not been interested in eating and tires very easily when he does try to breast-feed. His weight is down 5% from his birthweight and the remainder of his vital signs include a HR of 240, respiratory rate of 68, and oxygen saturation of 92%. His blood pressure is not obtained. Physical examination reveals a nondysmorphic newborn in moderate respiratory distress with subcostal retractions. Air entry throughout is good with bilateral basilar crackles. You appreciated a murmur heard best over the infant's back and left axilla. When you unwrap him, you note mottled legs with delayed capillary refill. You place him on a continuous cardiorespiratory monitor.

20. What is the next best step in his care?
     a. Obtain a chest x-ray
     b. Obtain a 12-lead ECG
     c. Obtain IV access
     d. Rapid sequence intubation

Stabilization of any critically ill patient requires first securing the ABCs. Currently, his airway is patent and although his breathing is labored, he remains stable with abnormally low, but acceptable oxygen saturations. Because supplemental oxygen can promote closing of the ductus arteriosus, it should be used with caution in any patient at risk of suffering from a ductal-dependent cardiac lesion. Next, consider the patient's circulation. He is mottled with delayed capillary refill and profound tachycardia. IV access must be obtained immediately, as this patient has evidence of circulatory collapse. Diagnostic studies, such as a chest x-ray, ECG, and echocardiogram will undoubtedly provide useful information, but they should not be performed until access is obtained.

21. You place an IV in his right arm and obtain blood samples to send to the laboratory. Which of the following laboratory values would be relevant to his care?
    a. CBC with differential
    b. Blood culture
    c. Electrolytes with blood urea nitrogen (BUN) and creatinine
    d. All of the above

This patient has tachycardia, respiratory distress, and poor perfusion. Overall, his picture is concerning for sepsis or congenital heart disease (CHD) but there should also be some consideration of congenital adrenal hyperplasia (CAH) which can present as shock in a newborn as well. Therefore, all of the above laboratory tests will be useful in differentiating the etiology of his shocklike condition.

22. What is your next management step while waiting for laboratory values to return?
    a. Obtain a chest x-ray
    b. Obtain a 12-lead ECG
    c. Administer prostaglandin infusion 0.05 mcg/kg/min
    d. Administer adenosine 0.1 mg/kg IV

Obtaining an ECG is the most appropriate next step. Adenosine is the treatment of choice for supraventricular tachycardia (SVT); The ECG will also provide you with useful information regarding the impulse vectors of the heart, which can be useful in distinguishing different congenital cardiac defects. An x-ray will also be helpful to further delineate the nature of his respiratory distress, and it would be most appropriate to call for a portable x-ray, as this patient is too ill to leave your immediate attention. Prostaglandin (PGE1) administration can be lifesaving in a newborn with ductal-dependent lesions and should therefore be considered in patients who presents in shock within the first several weeks of life. Prior to its administration, it is useful to gather as many clues as time allows to point you either away or toward a ductal-dependent cardiac lesion.

ECG reveals a normal axis, keeping in mind that right axis deviation is normal for a newborn. Chest x-ray shows cardiomegaly and lung fields that are hazy with increased vascular congestion. Your concern for cardiac disease is further heightened.

23. What additional physical exam finding could have provided you with a specific cardiac diagnosis in this patient?
    a. Hepatomegaly
    b. Absent femoral pulses
    c. Single second heart sound
    d. Preductal and postductal pulse-oximetry measurements
    e. All of the above

All of the above features of the physical examination are extremely important to note in a newborn; however, all but one are nonspecific findings. Hepatomegaly in this setting suggests heart failure, which can result from multiple etiologies. A single second heart sound is not specific for any one cardiac lesion. It merely suggests decreased blood flow across the pulmonic valve, which is seen in tetralogy of Fallot (TOF), tricuspid atresia, and pulmonic atresia. A preductal saturation 5% greater than postductal saturation suggests cardiac shunting across a patent ductus but is not specific for any one lesion. In contrast, absent or weak femoral pulses are a hallmark sign of coarctation of the aorta, as are decreased lower extremity blood pressures, and therefore should be considered diagnostic in an emergent setting in which an echocardiogram cannot be obtained.

24. With considerable evidence pointing toward the diagnosis of critical coarctation of the aorta, what is your next step in this patient's management?
    a. Administer furosemide (Lasix) 1 mg/kg IV
    b. Administer digoxin 20 mcg/kg IV

    c. Administer PGE1 infusion 0.05 mcg/kg/min

    d. Administer a 20 cc/kg NS bolus

Absent femoral pulses in a newborn who presents in shock is an indication for the immediate administration of PGE1. This patient also has signs of left heart failure and therefore would also benefit from Lasix and digoxin; however, PGE1 administration should take precedence. Because apnea is a well-known side effect of PGE1 infusion, you intubate the infant prior to starting the infusion. While preparing for intubation, the patient's heart rate climbs to near 300 bpm and you note very wide complexes on the monitor. The child is unresponsive and you cannot feel a femoral pulse on examination.

25.   What is your next step?

    a. Administer adenosine 0.1 mg/kg IV

    b. Administer amiodarone 5 mg/kg IV

    c. Cardiovert using 0.5 J/kg

    d. Defibrillate using 2 J/kg

The first step in management of pulseless VT is defibrillation with an initial dose of 2 J/kg with subsequent doses increased up to 4 J/kg. Synchronized cardioversion is performed when a pulse or signs of circulation are present. Adenosine is used to treat SVT, which is a narrow-complex tachycardia without P-waves. Amiodarone is an antiarrhythmic agent that can be used in both pulseless VT as well as VT with palpable pulses, but its administration should not precede defibrillation in this setting.

The patient's rhythm returns to a narrow-complex tachycardia at a rate of 220 bpm following the first defibrillation attempt. Next, you intubate and start PGE1. An echocardiogram is performed which confirms the suspected diagnosis and you initiate adjunctive therapy with Lasix and digoxin. The patient is transferred to the ICU for further stabilization prior to surgical correction.

Answers: 20-c, 21-d, 22-b, 23-b, 24-c, 25-d

CASE 6

You are working in the ED when Emergency Medical Services (EMS) brings in a 16-year-old girl for evaluation after a seizure. EMS reports that her parents heard "funny noises" coming from her room and found her lying on her bed in the midst of a generalized tonic-clonic seizure that lasted 60 seconds and resolved spontaneously. Her parents report that she has a history of depression but does not have a history of seizures. On arrival, her blood pressure is 140/70, her pulse is 120, respiratory rate 36, oxygen saturation of 100% on a nonrebreather (NRB) mask and temperature 37.5°C.

26.   What is your first step?

    a. ABCs, IV, oxygen, monitor

    b. Perform a complete physical examination

    c. Obtain more history from the parents and EMS if they are available

    d. Check a fingerstick blood glucose

All of these answers are appropriate for the case presented but remember to always start your evaluation of a potentially critically ill patient with the ABCs, establishing IV access, providing supplemental oxygen, and putting the patient on a cardiac monitor. This allows you to prepare for sudden deterioration and start following vital sign trends. In cases of altered mental status (AMS), the differential diagnosis is often very broad and little if any history can be garnered from the patient, making EMS, friends, and family valuable sources of potential clues to the etiology. Often the diagnosis can be made from a thorough physical examination. Checking a fingerstick glucose should be done early in the workup of AMS, especially in the setting of seizure. If there is no glucometer available, empiric treatment with IV dextrose is indicated. You place the patient on the monitor, establish IV access, document a normal blood sugar, and undress the patient to perform a physical examination. Your examination is notable for a Glasgow coma scale (GCS) of 11 with evidence of confusion but no focal weakness, a small occipital hematoma without step-off and well-healed superficial cuts on both wrists that her parents report were self inflicted during a particularly bad period of depression a year ago.

27. What is the next step?
    a. Obtain a head CT
    b. Send blood for serum and urine toxicologic screens, chemistries, CBC, and liver function tests
    c. Administer empiric antibiotics
    d. Perform a lumbar puncture (LP)

The workup for the patient with AMS often involves all of the above. After evaluating the ABCs, obtaining IV access, and placing the patient on the monitor, use elements of the history, vital signs and physical examination to try and narrow your differential diagnosis. This patient has a history of depression and past self-injurious behavior. Therefore, laboratory tests including toxicologic screen is indicated looking specifically for an anion gap, aspirin, acetaminophen, tricyclic antidepressants, and drugs of abuse.

She had a seizure and is now postictal. She is hypertensive, tachycardic, and tachypneic but without fever or hypoxia. She has evidence of head trauma on examination.

28. With this as a background, which of the following would be the most appropriate sequence of actions?
    a. IV antibiotics, head CT, LP if head CT normal
    b. ECG, IV fluids, head CT
    c. ECG, empiric activated charcoal, head CT
    d. IV antibiotics followed by LP

A "shotgun" approach is often taken with cases of AMS but this patient's history, vitals, and physical examination point to trauma or drug ingestion as the most likely culprits. Although meningitis or encephalitis should always be considered, the lack of fever, infectious prodrome, rash or meningismus make this somewhat less likely. An ECG is important to look for widened QRS complexes or (QT) prolongation, which would raise suspicion for tricyclic antidepressant overdose. In addition, salicylate and acetaminophen ingestions are relatively common and treatable. You whisk the patient off for head CT, which is normal, and while there, the nurse informs you that the laboratory just called with the following results:

Sodium 141 mEq/dL, potassium 4.0 mEq/dL, chloride 101 mEq/dL, bicarbonate 8 mEq/dL, BUN 20 mg/dL, creatinine 1.4 mg/dL, glucose 120 mg/dL

pH 7.2, Pco_2 20, PO_2 300, bicarbonate 8 mEq/dL

29. Which of the following ingestions is the most likely cause of the patient's symptoms?
    a. Acetaminophen
    b. Methylenedioxymethamphetamine MDMA (Ecstasy)
    c. Salicylates
    d. Methanol

The combination of the patient's presentation with seizures, tachycardia, and marked tachypnea with evidence of an anion gap metabolic acidosis combined with a respiratory alkalosis, make salicylates the most likely ingestion. Acetaminophen can cause massive hepatic necrosis if taken in large doses but is not known to cause seizures or acidosis unless a coingestant is present. MDMA is a club-drug that has been known to cause hyperthermia, tachycardia, hypertension, and seizures, usually in the setting of hyponatremia. Methanol can cause AMS, metabolic acidosis, and visual changes but is usually not associated with a respiratory alkalosis. The laboratory calls and informs you that the patient's salicylate level is 130 mg/dL.

30. How would you treat the patient's overdose?
   a. N-acetylcysteine orally
   b. Fomepizole
   c. 150 mEq/L of sodium bicarbonate IV
   d. Call the renal service for dialysis

Salicylate overdoses are common due to the fact that almost everyone has a bottle of aspirin in the medicine cabinet. Acute ingestion of salicylates can lead to vomiting, tinnitus, and AMS with a primary metabolic acidosis with a compensatory respiratory alkalosis picture on blood gas analysis. Metabolic acidosis is due to inhibition of oxidative phosphorylation in mitochondria leading to anaerobic metabolism while respiratory alkalosis is due to hyperventilation secondary to the acidosis. Significant ingestions can lead to seizures, coma, hyperthermia, and noncardiogenic pulmonary edema. Treatment involves alkalinizing the serum of patients in order to trap free salicylate in the urine for excretion. Dialysis is indicated for patients with an acute ingestion and levels >120 mg/dL, seizures, severe acidosis, coma, or pulmonary edema. N-acetylcysteine is the treatment for acetaminophen overdose while fomepizole is the antidote for toxic alcohols (methanol and ethylene glycol).

Answers: 26-a, 27-b, 28-c, 29-c, 30-c

CASE 7

An 18-day-old 4-kg baby boy is brought to your ED for evaluation of poor feeding. The 16-year-old mother reports that the child was a term product of a normal spontaneous vaginal delivery (NSVD) complicated by maternal fever requiring antibiotics. The baby was breast-feeding well until today when he seemed to be "out of breath" and he won't latch onto his mother's nipple. You eyeball the child and note a neonate with severe tachypnea and suprasternal and subcostal retractions.

31. What do you do?
   a. ABCs, IV, supplemental oxygen, and monitoring
   b. Administer albuterol via nebulizer
   c. Administer antibiotics
   d. Call for help

Although all of these interventions may be part of the resuscitation of this infant (especially calling for help), your first priority is a rapid assessment of the ABCs, obtaining IV access, and putting the patient on a monitor. Your quick assessment of this child is that he is in significant respiratory distress and respiratory distress often precedes circulatory collapse. You pull the code cart to the room, hook up the bag-valve mask (BVM), and obtain a complete set of vitals. The temperature is 39°C rectally, pulse 190, blood pressure 90/55, respiratory rate 90, and oxygen saturation 90% on room air. The child has an intact airway but has diffuse wheezing and very poor air movement bilaterally. He is tachycardic with some mottling of his extremities.

32. What should your next intervention be?
   a. Provide positive pressure with the BVM and 100% oxygen
   b. Give 20 cc/kg of NS IV
   c. Administer IV ampicillin and gentamicin
   d. Prepare for intubation

All four of these interventions are indicated in this patient. The infant is in the prearrest stage and needs immediate ventilatory support with 100% oxygen and positive pressure. A 20 cc/kg NS bolus is indicated for signs of poor perfusion and possible sepsis. Early initiation of antibiotic therapy is also critical. Preparations for intubation should be made as well in case the child does not improve soon. As you are working, you note that he is having episodes of apnea lasting 15 to 30 seconds associated with some dips in his HR to the 90s and desaturations.

33. Which of the following medications are you going to have at the bedside and ready?
    a. Epinephrine 0.1 mg/kg IV
    b. Epinephrine 0.01 mg/kg IV
    c. Atropine 0.02 mg/kg IV
    d. Vasopressin 0.4 to 1 unit/kg IV

First-line treatment for bradycardia associated with poor perfusion in a child of this age would be epinephrine 0.01 mg/kg IV. Higher-dose epinephrine is used if there is no IV access and the medication is to be given via the endotracheal tube (ETT) (0.1 mg/kg). Atropine is useful for bradycardia associated with excessive vagal tone, which is not the case in this scenario. Vasopressin is indicated as an option in pulseless arrest but does not have a role for bradycardia. You realize that the child's apnea and bradycardia mandate definitive control of the airway and begin preparations for intubation. As the nurse is drawing up rapid sequence intubation (RSI) medications, he suddenly stops breathing and turns blue. His HR drops into the 30s.

34. What is your next step?
    a. Start cardiopulmonary resuscitation (CPR)
    b. Immediately intubate the patient
    c. Give epinephrine IV
    d. Defibrillate at 2 J/kg

Once the child's HR drops below 60 bpm, chest compressions should be started. The child will need to be intubated and epinephrine may help increase the HR but your first job is to ensure adequate circulation to the heart and brain while these other maneuvers are accomplished. Defibrillation is indicated for pulseless rhythms such as VF or pulseless VT but is not indicated here. You begin chest compressions and BVM breaths and administer a dose of epinephrine. The HR promptly improves to 120 bpm and the child begins to have spontaneous, though ineffective ventilations.

35. Which of the following medications would be appropriate for induction and paralysis prior to intubation?
    a. Atropine, rocuronium, etomidate
    b. Succinylcholine, ketamine
    c. Succinylcholine, thiopental
    d. Lidocaine, vecuronium, etomidate

Remember your goals during RSI. You want to quickly render the patient unconscious and paralyze to achieve optimal intubating conditions without aspiration of stomach contents. All children less than 10 years of age should receive a dose of atropine prior to direct laryngoscopy to blunt the vagal surge that occurs during intubation. Succinylcholine, though not contraindicated in this case, should be given after atropine. Lidocaine is used in cases of increased ICP, which is not the case in this scenario. Thus, atropine, rocuronium, and etomidate constitute an appropriate regimen for RSI. You administer the medications and successfully intubate the patient using a Miller 1 blade and a 4.0 uncuffed ETT. You obtain a postintubation chest radiograph that reveals the ETT in good position and diffuse atelectasis with peribronchial cuffing and hyperinflation.

36. As the child is being wheeled to the ICU, a medical student who was observing the resuscitation asks what caused the infant's deterioration. How do you answer?
    a. Critical coarctation of the aorta with closure of the ductus arteriosus
    b. Bacterial sepsis
    c. Respiratory syncytial virus (RSV) infection with central apnea and respiratory failure
    d. Foreign body aspiration

Although all of these conditions can cause shock and/or respiratory distress, the combination of the child's age, the presence of fever and the chest radiograph findings are most consistent with RSV infection. RSV bronchiolitis is a significant cause of neonatal morbidity and typically presents with respiratory distress with or without fever. Neonates are particularly apt to develop apnea and bradycardia with RSV infection and the mechanism is thought to be one of central respiratory drive suppression. Coarctation of the aorta may present with shock but the presence of fever and the chest x-ray findings make this less common. Bacterial sepsis should always be a consideration in the critically-ill neonate and appropriate broad-spectrum antibiotic therapy initiated. Foreign body aspiration would be unlikely in this child due to the child's age and presence of fever.

Answers: 31-a, 32-a, 33-b, 34-a, 35-a, 36-c

CASE 8

You are out ice fishing on a frigid New England day when you hear screams coming from across the lake. You arrive to find a fellow fisherman dragging the limp, blue body of a 7-year-old boy from a hole in the ice. First responders report that he fell through a crack in the ice and was submerged for approximately 5 minutes. The water temperature under the ice is 5°C. You assess the child and note that he is not breathing but has a palpable pulse at a rate of 40.

37. A bystander is calling 911; what do you do?
    a. Begin rescue breathing
    b. Begin rescue breathing and chest compressions
    c. Gently remove the wet clothing and cover the child with blankets
    d. Perform abdominal thrusts to force the lake water from the child's lungs

Your first priority on arrival is to assess this child's ABCs. After you confirm that the child is unconscious, open his airway with a jaw thrust while maintaining in-line cervical spine immobilization (remember, he fell through the ice). If the child is not breathing, deliver two rescue breaths and then assess for signs of circulation. This child has bradycardia, but perfusing pulse rate of 40 bpm. Although normally pulse < 60 in a child of this age would prompt chest compressions, in a hypothermic arrest situation that may cause more harm than good. As the body cools, the basal metabolic needs decrease and an HR of 40, which under ordinary circumstances may not be adequate to meet the body's needs, may be sufficient. Plus, the hypothermic patient is at risk for spontaneous ventricular fibrillation (VF) below 28°C and chest compressions may turn a perfusing bradycardic rhythm into nonperfusing VF.

Removing wet clothing and preventing further heat loss is always a good idea, but should occur after assessment of the ABCs. Most hypothermic submersion victims are "dry-drowning" victims, where upon entering the water, they experience laryngospasm and little water enters the lungs, making abdominal thrusts unneeded and potentially harmful. You begin rescue breathing and EMS arrives. They immobilize the child and continue bagging him en route to the nearest hospital.

38. As you arrive at the ED, the child loses pulses and you see this rhythm (Figure A8-1) on the monitor; what do you do?

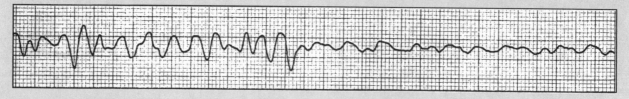

FIGURE A8-1 (From Senecal EL, Filbin MR. *Emergency Management of the Coding Patient: Cases, Algorithms, Evidence.* Malden, MA: Blackwell Publishing; 2005 with permission)

    a. Continue CPR
    b. Intubate the child without medications
    c. Establish IV access and administer epinephrine
    d. Defibrillate with 2 J/kg

This rhythm is VF and should be treated with immediate electricity! CPR, including ventilation and chest compressions, is appropriate to provide a means of oxygenation and cardiac output until the defibrillator is charged and ready to use. Attempts at IV access or intubation should never delay the delivery of defibrillation to a patient in VF. You deliver three stacked shocks of 2 J/kg, 2 to 4 J/kg, and 4 J/kg without return of pulses.

39. What should the next intervention be?
    a. Intubation and IV access while continuing CPR
    b. Continue CPR for 1 minute then reassess
    c. Deliver two rescue breaths via BVM
    d. Obtain a rectal temperature

During a pulseless arrest, after three stacked shocks are given in rapid succession, the patient should be intubated and have IV access obtained. In this patient, obtaining an accurate rectal temperature is also important and warming measures should be instituted. Malignant arrhythmias such as VF are often resistant to attempts at defibrillation or administration of epinephrine until the patient is warmed. You intubate the patient, continue CPR, and establish IV access, and document a rectal temperature of 28°C.

40. Which of the following is indicated next?
    a. Administration of 0.1 mg/kg of epinephrine via ETT followed by 30 to 60 seconds of CPR
    b. Administration of 0.01 mg/kg IV of epinephrine followed by 30 to 60 seconds of CPR
    c. Administration of bretylium followed by 30 to 60 seconds of CPR
    d. Administration of 4 to 10 units/kg of vasopressin followed by 30 to 60 seconds of CPR

After three stacked shocks, intubation, and IV access should occur followed by administration of a vasopressor such as epi-nephrine. The correct dose for epinephrine is 0.01 mg/kg IV. ETT administration of epinephrine is only indicated if IV access has not been established, and the dose would be ten times the IV dose. Vasopressin is an alternative to epinephrine in this case but the correct dose would be 0.4 to 1 units/kg. Bretylium was long considered the agent of choice for prophylaxis of VF in the set-ting of hypothermia. This recommendation was based on animal studies only and it was removed from both the Pediatric Advanced Life Support (PALS) and Advanced Cardiac Life Support (ACLS) algorithm in recent years due to decreased availability and the increased incidence of side effects, namely hypotension. You correctly administer 0.01 mg/kg of IV epinephrine fol-lowed by 30 to 60 seconds of CPR and then defibrillate again with 4 J/kg resulting in a perfusing rhythm with a rate of 90 bpm.

41. What is your next priority?
    a. Place a central venous catheter for central venous pressure monitoring
    b. Warm the patient with passive external warming
    c. Warm the patient with active external warming
    d. Warm the patient with active internal warming

With a core body temperature of 82°F, this patient qualifies as "severely hypothermic." Mild hypothermia is defined as a core temperature of > 32°C and is treated by removing wet clothes, providing a dry blanket and getting the patient out of the cold environment. This constitutes passive external rewarming and relies on the patient's own metabolic rate to warm. Moderate hypothermia, defined as a core temperature of 28°C to 32°C, is treated with passive external warming and active external warming. Examples of active external rewarming include heating blankets, radiant warmers, and hot packs. Consideration should also be given to active internal or core rewarming for the moderately hypothermic patient. Active internal rewarming is the most effective means to rapidly rewarm a patient and includes such modalities as cardiopulmonary bypass, extracorporeal life support with membrane oxygenation (ECMO), hemodialysis, pleural lavage, peritoneal lavage and often overlooked methods such as warmed, humidified oxygen and warmed IV fluids. You correctly determine that this child requires active internal warming and call the pediatric surgeons and ICU. The patient is successfully cannulated for ECMO and transported to the ICU.

Answers: 37-a, 38-d, 39-a, 40-b, 41-d

CASE 9

A 2-year-old boy presents to the ED at 5 a.m. for persistent cough. He began with a runny nose two nights ago and the cough has progressed since then. This evening he continued to cough and was unable to sleep. He has had no fevers, headache, vomiting or diarrhea, and no rash. In the past, he was hospitalized at 6 months of age for bronchiolitis that lasted 1 day. He has had a few episodes of wheezing in the past treated with a home nebulizer machine and albuterol. He lives at home with his parents and attends day care 3 days a week. There are no smokers in the home. He has been drinking normally and making wet diapers. On physical examination, you note a very dry, persistent cough. Vitals reveal a temperature of 98.6°F, HR of 106 bpm, respiratory rate of 24, blood pressure of 88/56, and oxygen saturation of 97%. He has clear nasal discharge. On lung examination, you hear some inspiratory stridor over the trachea and upper chest but no wheezes or crackles. He has no accessory muscle use. The remainder of the examination is normal.

42. What is the most likely diagnosis?
    a. Foreign body ingestion
    b. Croup
    c. Bronchiolitis
    d. Asthma
    e. Epiglottitis

The above patient presents with persistent cough worse at night and inspiratory stridor on examination, findings consistent with croup. Classically, the cough is described as a "barking seal." Foreign body should be considered in toddlers with respiratory symptoms as aspiration of small items is common. Objects can become lodged in the glottis, trachea, bronchi, or esophagus and cause cough or respiratory symptoms. Upper airway obstruction causes stridor, whereas lower obstruction causes wheeze; both may be associated with cough. Onset of symptoms, however, is usually acute, not over a few days as in this patient. Bronchiolitis presents with cough but usually has characteristic lung examination findings of coarse breath sounds and wheeze, which this patient does not have. Asthma also presents with cough but on lung examination presents with diminished air entry and wheeze. Finally, epiglottitis may present with stridor, but usually is accompanied by a high fever and a toxic appearance.

43. You note the patient has persistent cough and mild stridor. The parents ask what should be done next. What is the appropriate treatment for this child?
    a. Provide humidified oxygen
    b. Provide dexamethasone 0.6 mg/kg by mouth
    c. Order a CXR
    d. Encourage oral fluid intake

While it is important to remember to provide oxygen in patients with respiratory distress, this patient likely does not need it. He has normal respiratory effort and normal oxygenation. Humidified air may provide some relief for his cough, but he does not require supplemental oxygen. A CXR is not indicated in croup. If imaging is desired, soft tissue images of the neck are appropriate to visualize the glottis and subglottic space. Encouraging fluid intake is important to prevent dehydration and the patient has already been drinking well. The treatment of croup consists of steroids as they decrease inflammation; therefore, dexamethasone is the preferred choice. Oral, IM, and IV routes are equally efficacious.

The patient is given oral dexamethasone and sent home. Three days later, he presents back to the ED with persistent cough. The parents note that he did improve for about a day after the treatment, but over the past 24 hours he continues to cough and have noisy breathing. His vitals reveal a temperature of 99.4°F, HR of 108 bpm, respiratory rate of 28, and oxygen saturation of 97%. Persistent cough is present, although not as dry as previous. He continues to have clear nasal discharge. Lung examination reveals no appreciable stridor and diffuse expiratory wheezes. The remainder of the examination is normal.

44. What is the appropriate treatment for this child?
    a. Repeat dose of dexamethasone 0.6 mg/kg
    b. Start azithromycin to cover atypical pneumonia

c.   Try albuterol nebulizers and discharge with 5-day course of prednisolone

d.   Continue observation and supportive care

The patient now presents with continued cough and wheezing with resolution of stridor after a dose of steroids 3 days ago. His examination is most consistent with a viral-induced wheezing or asthma exacerbation, likely secondary to the movement of the virus causing croup to the lower airways, causing wheeze. A repeat dose of dexamethasone alone would be inappropriate, as the patient no longer has symptoms of croup. Steroids, however, are beneficial in asthma exacerbations and providing them along with a bronchodilator is beneficial. A 5-day course of a medium length-acting steroid such as prednisolone is appropriate. Observation and supportive care would be acceptable if the patient had no evidence of wheeze and no respiratory distress or if it was thought his symptoms were secondary to uncomplicated bronchiolitis. His history of prior wheezing episodes, however, suggests he requires treatment with steroids and a bronchodilator. An atypical or "walking" pneumonia can also cause cough and low-grade fevers and is typically caused by *Mycoplasma*. School age and teenage children are typically affected. Lung examination usually reveals diffuse crackles, which this patient does not have. For now, it appears appropriate to hold antibiotics.

The patient is given an albuterol nebulizer with resolution of his wheezing. He is given a first dose of oral prednisolone and observed for 3 hours without additional need for albuterol. He is sent home to finish 5 days of steroids and to give albuterol nebulizers every 4 hours. Two nights later, his parents return to the ED for persistent irritability and crying. He has continued with the runny nose and cough, although the cough has improved. They have been giving the prednisolone and albuterol as instructed. This evening he had a fever to 102°F for which they gave ibuprofen. On examination, his vitals reveal a temperature of 101.6°F, pulse 114, respiratory rate 24, and oxygen saturation 98%. Ear examination reveals red eardrums bilaterally, with the left containing fluid and a marked bulge and decreased movement with insufflation. Throat is clear and mucus membranes are moist. Lungs are clear bilaterally without stridor or wheeze. Heart is regular rate and rhythm, abdomen is soft and nontender. Extremities are warm and well-perfused without rash and capillary refill is < 2 seconds. Neurologic examination reveals an irritable but consolable child with no nuchal rigidity and normal strength, reflexes, and sensation.

45.   What is the most likely diagnosis?

a.   Bacteremia

b.   Urinary tract infection (UTI)

c.   Otitis media

d.   Pneumonia

e.   Meningitis

The patient now presents with irritability and fever in the setting of a known viral illness. Examination reveals a bulging, immobile and erythematous left tympanic membrane, consistent with otitis media. Upper respiratory infections are common antecedents to bacterial otitis media. Appropriate treatment consists of an antibiotic to cover *pneumococcus, Haemophilus influenzae*, and *Moraxella*. Amoxicillin is considered first-line therapy. Fever above 102°F (39°C) is considered significant for children 3 months to 36 months of age and deserves a thorough evaluation for SBI. Uncircumcised boys under 12 months of age have a significant risk of UTI. After that age, the risk of UTI is very low in boys. Bacteremia should be suspected in toxic-appearing children with significant fever without any localizing source of infection. Pneumonia is certainly a possibility in this patient with his history of respiratory symptoms but is effectively ruled out by his normal lung examination and lack of tachypnea. If a high suspicion cannot be confirmed by clinical examination, a chest x-ray would be indicated. Finally, fever and irritability can suggest meningitis, either viral or bacterial. Nuchal rigidity is a nonspecific finding and is not always present in meningitis. However, given his otherwise normal appearance, the most likely diagnosis is otitis media.

The patient is given a dose of acetaminophen and amoxicillin. He is observed to be drinking normally and have normal interactions with his parents. He is discharged home with a 10-day course of antibiotics and fever control. On follow-up with his pediatrician 48 hours later, he is well appearing and afebrile. Examination reveals a healing otitis media and is otherwise normal. Follow-up is scheduled for 4 weeks for an ear reassessment for resolution.

Answers: 42-b, 43-b, 44-c, 45-c

CASE 10

You receive a page to labor and delivery (L&D) for a vaginal delivery of a premature infant. The mother is gravida 3, para 1 (G3P1) with a prior miscarriage. Her current pregnancy is at 31 weeks and has been uneventful. On the day of presentation, she began to develop contractions. In L&D upon arrival, her cervix was already 4 cm and effaced, and shortly thereafter she had a gush of vaginal fluid that was meconium stained. Tocometry showed a fetal HR initially of 140 with good beat-to-beat variability. Her contractions increased in frequency and the cervix became fully dilated. As she was pushing to deliver, the baby's HR developed late-decelerations to 110, followed by frank bradycardia to 90.

46. What is the foremost consideration as this baby is delivered?
    a. Rapid drying and warming
    b. Administration of blow-by oxygen
    c. Suction of oropharynx after delivery of head but before delivery of shoulders
    d. Availability of epinephrine to administer endotracheally

The first priority in resuscitating a newborn through meconium is to suction the oropharynx and nares before delivery of the shoulders. Meconium is a noxious substance that if aspirated into the newborn's lungs can result in meconium aspiration syndrome (MAS). This is essentially a chemical pneumonitis that causes alveolar damage, exudates, and respiratory distress in the newborn. It is important to suction before delivery of the shoulders because first-time expansion of the newborn's chest causes intrathoracic negative pressure to suck contents of the oropharynx into the trachea.

Thorough suctioning is done prior to delivering the shoulders. The baby is delivered completely without incident; however, the newborn is limp and making no respiratory effort.

47. What is the next priority?
    a. Dry, position, and stimulate the baby
    b. Immediate orotracheal intubation followed by deep suctioning
    c. Laryngoscopy with deep tracheal suctioning
    d. Positive-pressure ventilation (PPV) with a BVM

Routine steps in the care of a newborn typically begin with drying and warming the baby, proper positioning (i.e., supine, slight downward head tilt), mouth/nose suctioning, and stimulation to breathe. This of course changes in the presence of meconium. In that case, the first step depends on how the baby looks upon delivery. The three important signs to evaluate are respiratory effort, muscle tone, and HR. A vigorous child has adequate respiratory effort, good muscle tone, and a 9 HR >100. If this is the case, routine neonatal care can proceed. If not, then laryngoscopy is indicated with deep tracheal suctioning of meconium-stained secretions, as well as suctioning of the hypopharynx. This should be repeated if a large amount of meconium is suctioned from the trachea. It is important to note here that there is a move afoot in the literature and in practice to go away from deep tracheal suctioning with laryngoscopy in this setting. Preliminary data shows that this may not add benefit over oropharyngeal suctioning followed by BVM ventilation alone.

Deep suctioning with laryngoscopy is done with return of a moderate amount of meconium, and this is repeated with return of a smaller amount. The baby gasps for the first breath and continues with shallow, gasping breaths. She has blue extremities as well as blue lips.

48. What is the next step in her management?
    a. BVM ventilation at 40 to 60 per minute
    b. Intubate and administer epinephrine 0.1 mg/kg OT
    c. Intubate and start CPR
    d. Start CPR if HR is <100

At this point in the management of the newborn with meconium, after deep tracheal suctioning, an assessment is made whether PPV is needed. Indications include gasping breaths or apnea, central cyanosis, or an HR <100. This baby meets these criteria. Newborns are relatively easy to bag-mask-ventilate, and this skill should be foremost in your repertoire, as it is the most effective means of resuscitating the newborn in distress. Neither intubation nor CPR is indicated at this point, as the vast majority of newborns will respond to PPV alone. This allows collapsed alveoli to expand and for gas exchange to occur.

PPV is performed with a BVM apparatus for 30 seconds and the newborn is reassessed. His breathing seems more effective and his perioral cyanosis seems to have improved. You feel his umbilical pulse at about 90 per minute.

49. What do you do now?
    a. Intubate and give epinephrine 0.1 mg/kg ETT
    b. Start CPR
    c. Continue blow-by oxygen and start umbilical vein access
    d. Continue BVM ventilation alone

In a newborn who requires PPV (i.e., gasping/apnea, central cyanosis, HR <100), BVM ventilation is done for 30 seconds followed by reassessment as above. If the child is breathing adequately and has an HR >100, then routine postpartum care can be initiated. If the HR is <100, then BVM ventilation must resume for another 30 seconds.

50. The baby is then bagged for another 30 seconds and the HR is now 60 bpm. What should be the next action?
    a. Intubation, epinephrine, and CPR
    b. Continue BVM ventilation alone
    c. Intubation and atropine per ETT
    d. Continue BVM and start CPR

The threshold for starting CPR is Pulse < 60 per minute. Intubation is still not indicated until CPR is performed with BVM ventilations for another 30 seconds and the newborn is reassessed. If this is not successful, intubation should be performed while CPR is ongoing; and if the HR remains < 60 per minute, epinephrine 0.1 mg/kg ETT should be administered. In the meantime, IV access should be attempted. Umbilical vein access is somewhat time-consuming, while scalp or extremity veins are relatively easy to cannulate in the newborn. If IV access is secured, then epinephrine 0.01 mg/kg can be administered.

This baby is intubated as CPR is ongoing. More meconium is suctioned from the trachea and epinephrine 0.1 mg/kg via ETT is administered. Ventilation and CPR are continued for another 30 seconds and paused for reassessment. The HR is now 120 per minute and her face looks a bit pinker. A scalp vein is cannulated and she is administered a 10 cc/kg bolus of NS. She is transferred to the NICU where she remains intubated for another day before she is able to breathe on her own.

Answers: 46-c, 47-c, 48-a, 49-d, 50-d

Common Drugs

Drug	Indication	Mechanism	Dose	Subsequent doses	Notes
Adenosine	Stable narrow-complex tachycardia	AV nodal blocker	0.1 mg/kg IV push max 6 mg	0.2 mg/kg IV push max 12 mg	Rapid bolus technique
Albuterol	Bronchospasm	β_2-agonist	0.15 mg/kg nebulized over 10 to 20 min (max 5 mg) 90 µg/puff MDI 1 to 2 puffs	May use continuous nebulized albuterol in cases of severe bronchospasm	Continuous use may cause tachycardia, hypokalemia
	Hyperkalemia	β_2-agonist shifts potassium into cells	0.15 mg/kg nebulized	q15min	
Alprostadil (PGE1)	Ductal-dependent cardiac disease	Vasodilator, maintains patency of ductus arteriosus	0.05 to 0.1 mcg/kg/min	Titrate to clinical response 0.01 to 0.4 mcg/kg/min	
Amiodarone	For refractory pulseless VT/VF	Class III antiarrhythmic	5 mg/kg IV/IO push		Max 15 mg/kg/day
	Stable VT	Class III antiarrhythmic	5 mg/kg IV/IO over 20 to 60 min		
Aminophylline (theophylline is 80% aminophylline)	Bronchospasm	PDE inhibitor	IV load 6 mg/kg	Continuous 1 mg/kg/h	Goal therapeutic level 5–15 µg/ml Toxicity includes GI upset, seizures, and arrhythmias
Atropine	Bradycardia	Muscarinic receptor blocker (anticholinergic)	0.02 mg/kg IV push min 0.1 mg max 1 mg	May repeat × 1	
Calcium chloride	Hyperkalemia, calcium-channel blocker overdose	Stabilizes cardiac myocyte cell membranes	20 mg/kg IV/IO (0.2 mL/kg of 10% solution)		
Calcium gluconate	Hyperkalemia	Stabilizes cardiac myocyte cell membranes	100 mg/kg IV/IO (1 mL/kg) of 10% solution		

Drug	Indication	Mechanism	Dose	Subsequent doses	Notes
Diazepam (Valium)	Seizure	Benzodiazepine, promotes GABAergic transmission	0.1 to 0.3 mg/kg IV (max dose 10 mg) 0.5 mg/kg PR (max dose 20 mg)		Beware of respiratory depression and need for emergent airway management
Diphenhydramine (Benadryl)	Allergy/anaphylaxis	H_1-receptor blocker	1.25 mg/kg IV/IM max 50 mg	q6h	
Dopamine	Hypotension/shock	Vasopressor: renal dopamine receptors stimulated at low dose (1 to 5 mcg/kg/min); beta-receptors stimulated at moderate dose (5 to 10 mcg/kg/min); alpha-receptors stimulated at high dose (10 to 20 mcg/kg/min)	1 to 20 mcg/kg/min IV infusion		
Dobutamine	Hypotension/shock	Vasopressor (β_1 - >β_2-agonist)	2 to 20 mcg/kg/min IV infusion		Causes peripheral vasodilation which may result in hypotension
Epinephrine	Asystole/PEA	Sympathomimetic (α_1-, α_2-, β_1-, and β_2-agonist)	0.01 mg/kg IV/IO (1:10,000, 0.1 mL/kg) 0.1 mg/kg ETT (1:1,000, 0.1 mL/kg)	Repeat q3 to 5 min during CPR	
	Pulseless VT/VF	Sympathomimetic (α_1-, α_2-, β_1-, and β_2-agonist)	0.01 mg/kg IV/IO (1:10,000, 0.1 mL/kg) 0.1 mg/kg ETT (1:1,000, 0.1 mL/kg)	Repeat q3 to 5 min during CPR	
	Bradycardia	Sympathomimetic (α_1-, α_2-, β_1-, and β_2-agonist)	0.01 mg/kg IV/IO (1:10,000, 0.1 mL/kg) 0.1 mg/kg ETT (1:1,000, 0.1 mL/kg)	Repeat q3 to 5 min	
	Hypotension/shock	Sympathomimetic (α_1-, α_2-, β_1-, and β_2-agonist)	0.1 to 1 mcg/kg/min IV infusion	Titrate to effect	Tachycardia, hypertension, arrhythmia, nausea, and vomiting
	Anaphylaxis	Sympathomimetic (α_1-, α_2-, β_1-, and β_2-agonist)	0.01 mg/kg SQ/IM max 0.3 to 0.5 mg (1:1,000, 0.1 mL/kg)	May repeat SQ/IM dose q20min or in adults 100 mcg IV over 5 to 10 min (100 mcg = 1 mL of 1:10,000 solution dissolved in 9 mL NS)	EpiPen Jr 0.15 mg EpiPen 0.3 mg

Drug	Indication	Mechanism	Dose	Subsequent doses	Notes
	Bronchospasm	Sympathomimetic (α_1-, α_2-, β_1-, and beta-1-, and beta-2-agonist)	SQ 0.01 mL/kg (max 0.3 mL)	Repeat q20min × three doses	Rarely used
Epinephrine (racemic 2.25%)	Upper airway obstruction; bronchospasm	Sympathomimetic (α_1-, α_2-, β_1-, and β_2-agonist)	0.05 mL/kg in 3 mL NS over 20 min max 0.5 mL	Repeat as needed	
L-Epinephrine (1:1,000)	Upper airway obstruction; bronchospasm	Sympathomimetic (α_1-, α_2-, β_1-, and β_2-agonist)	0.5 mL/kg in 3 mL NS max: <4 yo: 2.5 mL >4yo: 5 mL	Repeat as needed	
Fentanyl	Conscious sedation for electrical cardioversion	Opiate and sympathetic blocker	50 to 100 mcg IV bolus	Repeat q5 to 20 min as needed	Typically used in conjunction with benzodiazepines; Beware of respiratory depression and need for airway emergent management
Fosphenytoin	Seizure/status epilepticus	Multifactorial, primarily sodium channel blocker	20 mg PE/kg IV at max rate of 3 mg PE/kg/min		Dosed as phenytoin equivalents (PE). May cause hypotension
Furosemide (Lasix)	Hyperkalemia	Diuretic	20 to 80 mg IV (higher doses for patients already on Lasix)	Repeat q2 to 6 h	
Glucose	Altered mental status/hypoglycemia	Cellular energy source	0.5 to 1 g/kg IV/IO 2 to 4 mL/kg of D25 5 to 10 mL/kg of D10 10 to 20 mL/kg of D5	Repeat as needed	Given empirically to patients with altered mental status if the blood glucose level is unknown
Insulin (regular)	Hyperkalemia	Shifts potassium into cells	0.1 unit/kg IV/IO		
Ipratropium (Atrovent)	Bronchospasm	Antimuscarinic causing smooth muscle relaxation	<12 yo: 250 µg >12 yo: 500 µg nebulized over 10 to 20 min 18 µg/puff aerosol: 1 to 2 puffs	Repeat q4 to 6 h	Combination with albuterol in asthma ("stacked" 3 treatments). Do not use aerosol in peanut or soy allergy

Drug	Indication	Mechanism	Dose	Subsequent doses	Notes
Kayexalate (sodium polystyrene sulfonate)	Hyperkalemia	Cation exchange resin	15 to 60 g PO or PR	Repeat in 60 min	
Lidocaine	VF/stable VT/pulseless VT	Class I antiarrhythmic	1 mg/kg IV/IO	1 mg/kg/min IV drip	
Lorazepam (Ativan)	Seizure/status epilepticus	Benzodiazepine, promotes GABAergic transmission	0.1 mg/kg IV max dose 4 mg	Repeat q3 to 5 min	Beware of respiratory depression and need for emergent airway management
Magnesium sulfate	Torsades de pointes	Unclear mechanism; possible calcium antagonist	25 mg/kg IV/IO		
	Bronchospasm	Unclear mechanism; possible calcium antagonist	IV 25 to 75 mg/kg (max 2 g) over 20 min	May repeat q4 to 6 h	May cause muscle weakness, respiratory depression
Mannitol	Head injury	Osmotic diuretic	0.5 to 1 g/kg IV		May cause hypotension
Methylprednisolone (Solu-Medrol)	Bronchospasm/ allergy/anaphylaxis	Anti-inflammatory	0.5 to 1 mg/kg IV	q6 to 12 h	
Milrinone	Inotropic therapy	Phosphodiesterase inhibitor	50 mcg/kg IV bolus over 5 to 15 min	Continuous infusion 0.5 to 1 mcg/kg/min	May cause hypotension
Naloxone (Narcan)	Altered mental status or suspected opiate overdose	Opioid mu receptor blocker	0.1 mg/kg IV/ETT	Repeat as needed q3min	Smaller doses may be used to reverse sedation
Norepinephrine (Levophed)	Hypotension/shock	Vasopressor (α_1-, α_2-, and β_1-agonist)	0.05 to 2 mcg/kg/min IV infusion		Primarily stimulates alpha-receptors to cause vasoconstriction
Pentobarbital	Refractory seizure	Barbiturate, promotes GABAergic transmission and induces coma	10 to 15 mg/kg over 1 h	Continuous infusion of 1 to 3 mg/kg/h	Requires intubation
Phenylephrine (Neo-Synephrine)	Hypotension/shock	Vasopressor (α_1-, α_2-agonist)	0.1 to 0.5 mcg/kg/ min IV infusion 5 to 20 mcg/kg bolus q10 to 15 min		

Drug	Indication	Mechanism	Dose	Subsequent doses	Notes
Phenobarbital	Status epilepticus	Barbiturate, promotes GABAergic transmission	Load 20 mg/kg IV at max rate 1 mg/kg/min		Beware of respiratory depression and need for emergent airway management
Phenytoin (Dilantin)	Seizure/status epilepticus	Sodium channel blocker; cell membrane stabilizer	Load 20 mg/kg IV at max rate 1 mg/kg/min		May cause hypotension, bradycardia
Prednisone	Bronchospasm	Anti-inflammatory	1 to 2 mg/kg PO	q12 to 24 h	See methylprednisolone for IV
	Allergy/anaphylaxis	Anti-inflammatory	1 to 2 mg/kg PO	q12 to 24 h	See methylprednisolone for IV
Prednisolone	Bronchospasm	Anti-inflammatory	1 to 2 mg/kg PO	q12 to 24 h	See methylprednisolone for IV
Procainamide	VT	Class I antiarrhythmic	15 mg/kg IV/IO over 30 to 60 min		Do not administer with amiodarone
Ranitidine	Allergy/anaphylaxis	H_2-receptor blocker	1 mg/kg IV max 50 mg	q8h	
Sodium bicarbonate	Hyperkalemia	Shifts potassium into cells	1 mEq/kg IV/IO bolus	Repeat in 15 to 60 min if needed	Infuse slowly and only with adequate ventilation
	Neonatal acidosis		2 mEq/kg or 4 mL/kg of 4.2% solution		Slowly through umbilical vein
Terbutaline	Bronchospasm	β-receptor agonist	IV load 10 µg/kg; SQ 0.01 mL/kg (max 0.3 mL)	IV continuous 0.1 to 4.0 µg/kg/min	May repeat SQ dose q20min × 3
Valproic acid	Status epilepticus	Promotes GABAergic transmission	15 to 20 mg/kg IV max rate 20 mg/min		

Intubation drugs

Drug	Indication	Mechanism	Dose	Benefits	Risks
Adjuvant					
Lidocaine	in head injury	Unclear mechanism	1 mg/kg IV	Blunt increase in ICP. Prevents bronchospasm	
Atropine	Pretreatment for intubation	Muscarinic receptor blockade	0.02 mg/kg IV push min 0.1 mg max 1 mg	Blunts Vaga effect of laryngoscopy	
Vecuronium, rocuronium, pancuronium	Pretreatment for intubation	Nondepolarizing neuromuscular blocker	One-tenth normal dose	Blunt increase in ICP with succinylcholine	
Fentanyl	Pretreatment for intubation	Opiate	1 to 2 mcg/kg IV	Blunts sympathetic response to intubation	
Sedative/Hypnotic					
Midazolam (Versed)	Sedation	Benzodiazepine	0.05 to 0.1 mg/kg IV	Anticonvulsant properties, rapid onset	Hypotension
Fentanyl	Analgesic	Opiate	1 to 4 mcg/kg IV	Fewest hemodynamic effects	Chest wall rigidity with rapid administration
Etomidate	Sedation	Imidazole	0.1 to 0.3 mg/kg IV	Hemodynamically stable, cerebroprotective	Adrenal suppression with continuous infusion
Ketamine	Sedation	Dissociative amnestic	1 to 4 mg/kg IV	Augments HR and BP, bronchodilator	Increases ICP, HR and BP response
Propofol	Sedation	Phenolic	1 to 3 mg/kg IV	Rapid onset	Hypotension
Thiopental	Sedation	Barbiturate	1 to 5 mg/kg IV	Cerebroprotective, rapid onset, brief duration of action	Hypotension
Paralyzing agent					
Vecuronium	Paralysis	Nondepolarizing neuromuscular blocker	0.1 to 0.2 mg/kg IV		Prolonged paralysis (45–60 min) compared with rocuronium or succinylcholine
Rocuronium	Paralysis	Nondepolarizing neuromuscular blocker	0.6 to 1.2 mg/kg IV	Rapid acting, fewer side effects than succinylcholine	Prolonged paralysis (20–30 min) compared with succinylcholine
Succinylcholine	Paralysis	Depolarizing neuromuscular blocker	1 to 2 mg/kg IV	Rapid onset of paralysis, rapid recovery (10 min)	Hyperkalemia, Bradycardia, Malignant Hyperthermia, Hyperthermia, Trismus

AV, atrioventricular; IV, intravenous; MDI, metered-dose inhaler; q, every; PGE1, prostaglandin E_1; VT, ventricular tachycardia; VF, ventricular fibrillation; IO, intraosseous; PDE, phosphodiesterase; GABA, gamma-aminobutyric acid; PR, per rectum; PEA, pulseless electrical activity; CPR, cardiopulmonary resuscitation; ETT, endotracheal tube; SQ, subcutaneous; IM, intramuscular; NS, normal saline; yo; years old; PE, phenytoin equivalent; D25, 25% dextrose in water; D10, 10% dextrose in water; D5, 5% dextrose in water; PO, per os; ICP, intracranial pressure; BP, blood pressure; HR, heart rate.

Important Formulas

ETT size	< 28 weeks gestational age	2.5 uncuffed
	28 to 32 weeks gestational age	3.0 uncuffed
	> 32 weeks gestational age	3.5 uncuffed
	Term-adolescent	Age (years)/4 + 4
Tip to lip distance	< 44 weeks gestational age (< 1 month)	6 + weight (kg)
	> 44 weeks gestational age (> 1 month)	$3 \times$ ETT size
Oro/Nasogastric tube size	$2 \times$ ETT size	
Hypotension	70 mm Hg + (age in years $\times$ 2) = 5th %tile for systolic blood pressure	

Index

Note: Page numbers in italic indicate figures; page numbers followed by *t* indicate tables.